CARBOPHOBIA

CARBOPHOBIA

THE SCARY TRUTH
ABOUT AMERICA'S
LOW-CARB CRAZE

....

MICHAEL GREGER, MD

Lantern Books • New York

A Division of Booklight Inc.

2005
Lantern Books
One Union Square West, Suite 201
New York, NY 10003

Printed in the United States of America

Library of Congress Cataloging-in-Publication Data

Greger, Michael.
Carbophobia : the scary truth about America's low-carb craze / by Michael Greger.
p. cm.
Includes bibliographical references.
ISBN 1-59056-086-8 (alk. paper)
1. Low-carbohydrate diet. 2. Reducing diets. I. Title.
RM237.73.G74 2005
613.2'83—dc22
2004025929

*Dedicated to the memory
of Rachel Elizabeth Huskey*

TABLE OF CONTENTS

INTRODUCTION

DO YOU REMEMBER WHEN DR. ATKINS' DIET BOOK BROKE publishing records, selling over 100,000 copies a month and shooting to the top of the bestseller charts? Atkins became a media darling and did dozens of print, radio and television interviews a week. All across the country, people were reading his book. The year was 1972.

You may also recall that, the year after *Dr. Atkins' Diet Revolution* was first published, Dr. Atkins was brought before a Senate investigation on diet fads and frauds. At the congressional inquiry the head of the American Medical Association (AMA)'s nutrition council called the Atkins Diet a "serious threat to health," and the founder and chair of Harvard's nutrition department for 34 years went on record calling for Dr. Atkins to be brought up on malpractice charges for writing what he called such "dangerous nonsense." The president of the American College of Nutrition at the time declared, "Of all the bizarre diets that have been proposed in the last 50 years, this is the most dangerous to the public if followed for any length of time."

By the late '70s, diet rival Nathan Pritikin, who advocated a low-fat, plant-based diet after claiming it had reversed his own heart disease, locked horns with Atkins in nationally televised debates. The public started questioning the Atkins Diet, and Atkins' medical practice started to suffer. Fearing, in his own words, that Pritikin had begun "to be listened to," Atkins filed a $5 million lawsuit, charging Pritikin with slander. When Pritikin tragically lost his 28-year battle with radiation-induced leukemia, Dr. Atkins reportedly continued his lawsuit against Pritikin's grieving widow.

Before he died, however, Pritikin directed that his body be autopsied. He wanted to show the world what his diet could do. The autopsy findings were published in the *New England Journal of Medicine* in an article entitled "Nathan Pritikin's heart." Evidently, his arteries were as "soft and pliable" as a teenager's, with no signs of heart disease. "In a man 69 years old," wrote the pathologist, "the near absence of atherosclerosis and the complete absence of its effects are remarkable."

In contrast, according to a medical examiner's report at the time of his death in 2003, Dr. Atkins was overweight and stricken with hypertension and heart disease—all conditions Atkins claimed his diet would cure. Although Atkins' health may indeed be a matter of legitimate public concern, more troubling is whether or not the Atkins Corporation lied to the American public to shield their assets.

When Atkins suffered a cardiac arrest and nearly died in 2002, the Atkins Corporation quickly posted a statement on its website emphatically denying that the event had anything to do with his diet. "Clearly," the statement read, "his own nutritional protocols have left him, at the age of 71, with an extraordinarily healthy cardiovascular system." Atkins himself went on television the week after his cardiac arrest, categorically denying he had had any blockages of his coronary arteries. "So what are they [my critics] going to say," he boasted to Katie Couric, "now that they know I don't have any blockages?"

Of course he did have blockages. His cardiologist has divulged that indeed Atkins' coronary arteries were "perhaps 30 to 40% blocked," a fact even his widow was forced to acknowledge. After the coroner's report on Atkins' death was leaked, Veronica Atkins went from swearing on *Larry King Live* that her husband did *not* have coronary artery disease to finally admitting that his cardiovascular system may not have been as fit as the public had been led to believe. "Robert did have some progression of his coronary artery disease in the last three years of his life," she finally admitted in a public statement, "including some new blockage of a secondary artery. . . ." This suggests, as a former director of the U.S. National Institutes of Health accused, that "Dr. Atkins wasn't being straightforward with his patients, with the public."

Dr. Atkins died in 2003, but with billion-dollar backers, his diet didn't die with him. Millions of Americans continue to risk their health on Atkins-like diets. It seems everywhere one goes these days, the Atkins "A" can be found. In the first six months of 2004, no fewer than 1,864 new "low-carb" products were launched. Now there is everything from low-carb bread to low-carb gummy bears. Hershey's and Nestle are making low-carb candy bars, and Coke and Pepsi have launched carb-cutting colas. Kellogg's even defrosted some of its flakes and premiered a reduced-carb version of Fruit Loops. Krispy Kreme has a lower-carb doughnut in the works, and, thanks in part to pork-rind sales, hog prices are at record highs. All of this has public health experts very concerned.

The official condemnations of the Atkins Diet from the medical authorities of the '70s continue to hold weight to this day. The Atkins Corporation claims that the basic tenets of the Atkins Diet have remained "consistent since 1972," insisting that "nothing in the earlier books is wrong." But public health experts are no less troubled now than when the fad struck 30 years ago.

Warnings from medical authorities continue to pour in. "People need to wake up to the reality," writes former U.S. Surgeon General C. Everett Koop, that the Atkins Diet is "unhealthy and can be dangerous." The largest organization of food and nutrition professionals in the world calls the Atkins Diet "a nightmare of a diet." The official spokesperson of the American Dietetic Association (ADA) elaborated: "The Atkins Diet and its ilk—any eating regimen that encourages gorging on bacon, cream, and butter while shunning apples, all in the name of weight loss—are a dietitian's nightmare." The ADA has been warning Americans about the potential hazards of the Atkins Diet for almost 30 years now.

Dr. Atkins dismissed such criticism as "dietitian talk." "My English sheepdog," Atkins once said, "will figure out nutrition before the dieticians do." The problem for Atkins (and his sheepdog) is that the National Academy of Sciences, the most prestigious scientific body in the United States, agrees with the AMA and the ADA in opposing the Atkins Diet. So do the American Cancer Society, the American Heart Association, the Cleveland Clinic, Johns Hopkins University, the American Kidney Fund, the American College of Sports Medicine, and the National Institutes of Health. In fact, there does not seem to be a single major governmental or nonprofit medical, nutrition, or science-based organization in the world that supports the Atkins Diet. As a 2004 medical journal review concluded, the Atkins Diet "runs counter to all the current evidence-based dietary recommendations."

This book is not just some other diet doctor's pronouncement. This is not the Dr. Greger Diet versus the Dr. Atkins Diet. This is a century of medical science versus the Atkins Diet. This is not a case of academic "he said/she said." This is a case of a multi-billion-dollar corporation with a financial stake in ignoring "all the current evidence-based dietary recommendations," no matter what the human cost.

You don't have to take my word for it. If this book doesn't convince you, go to www.AtkinsExposed.org and read the American Medical Association's scathing official critique yourself. Read what the founder of the Harvard Nutrition Department, and the current chair, have to say about the Atkins Diet. Posted free online at AtkinsExposed.org are dozens of full-text official position statements and journal articles from medical and nutrition authorities across the country, warning of the widespread potential risks of low-carb diets.

This book is a summary of their findings (all supported by the reference section in the back, which I invite you to consult as you read). As Chapter 1 explains, in light of the evidence the Atkins Diet seems nothing more than a "modern twist on an antique food fad." Chapter 2 exposes the "factually flawed" science underlying the theories and arguments of popular low-carbohydrate diets and addresses the real reasons why the United States now has the most obese population on earth. Chapter 3 questions the effectiveness of low-carb diets when it comes to weight loss, demonstrating that every single study lasting more than six months found that the Atkins Diet failed to show any significant advantage over the very same high-carbohydrate diets that Dr. Atkins blamed for our epidemic of obesity.

The fourth chapter covers the short-term side effects of the diet, warning of the potential harm inherent in the metabolically deranged state of ketosis, for which every Atkins dieter strives. Chapter 5 documents the expected long-term consequences of following a diet that restricts fruits and vegetables but encourages the intake of saturated animal fat and protein. It also tells the story of Rachel Elizabeth Huskey, a Missouri teen who could very well have been killed by the Atkins Diet. The final chapter offers a safe and effective alternative to low-carb diets.

Finally, the addendum gives the Atkins Corporation a chance to present its side. Within weeks of launching my website I received a hostile letter from the corporation's lawyers threatening to sue me for speaking out about the dangers associated with its diet. I've posted the letter and my response in its entirety at www.AtkinsExposed.org but have included the major points at the end of this book.

A 2003 review of low carb "theories" in the *Journal of the American College of Nutrition* concluded that "Carbophobia is a form of nutritional misinformation infused into the American psyche through . . . advertising . . . infomercials . . . and best-selling diet books." By countering this misinformation with scientific fact, I hope to give the public the tools with which to make up their own minds.

CHAPTER ONE

ANTIQUE FOOD FAD

·····················

DR. ATKINS HAD A DREAM

THERE IS NOTHING NEW OR REVOLUTIONARY ABOUT LOW-CARB diets. Many types have been peddled under various names for over a hundred years, but, "By whatever name," one nutrition textbook reads, "the diet is to be avoided."

In 1864, an English undertaker and coffin maker by the name of William Banting wrote a book called *Letter on Corpulence* that advocated four meals per day of meat or fish and "scrupulous" avoidance of "starchy or saccharine matter." Based on what we know now about these diets, Banting's book may very well have added to Banting's business.

After apparently failing to produce the promised sustained weight loss, the high-fat fad melted away, only to re-emerge in the 1920s with a doctor advocating a minimum of three porterhouse steaks a day and stating that the only two perfect foods were probably "fresh fat meat and water." It then disappeared until the 1940s when a book appeared extolling the virtues of eating whale blubber. It was recycled again in the 1960s with Dr. Herman Taller's bestseller *Calories Don't Count*, which discouraged people from exercising. Taller's diet empire collapsed when he was found guilty of six counts of mail fraud for using the book to promote a particular brand of safflower capsules, which the court called a "worthless scheme foisted on a gullible public." That same year, Dr. Irwin Stillman wrote the *Doctor's Quick Weight Loss Diet*, allowing his patients to eat only meat, eggs, and cheese. Stillman himself died of a heart attack, but not before misleading 20 million people onto his diet.

One might wonder why, if this kind of diet was the "ultimate," "foolproof" path to "permanent joyful weight loss" that "WORKS 100% OF THE TIME!" (emphasis in original), it always seemed to quickly fade into obscurity, only to be resurrected shortly afterward by publishers guaranteed a new bestseller by America's short attention span. This brings us to 1972 and the publication of *Dr. Atkins' Diet Revolution*.

The Atkins Diet was centered on fried pork rinds, heavy cream, cheese, and meat. For Atkins, bacon and butter were health foods and bread and bananas were "poison."

Drawing on his experience as a salesman and resort entertainer, Atkins proved a natural at self-promotion. He was featured in *Vogue* magazine (in fact, the Atkins Diet was first known as the "Vogue Diet") and soon after appeared on the *Tonight Show* and *The Merv Griffin Show*. In 1973, the publisher boasted that Atkins' book was the "fastest selling book in publishing history."

The final chapter of *Dr. Atkins' Diet Revolution* was entitled "Why We Need a Revolution. . . ." It detailed his proposal to have some carbs literally banned. "Our laws must be changed," Atkins declared, "to provide a proper way of eating for everyone." He urged everyone to start lobbying their legislators. "Political action and protest on your part," he wrote, "can help revolutionize the food industry by forcing it to decarbohydratize many foods . . . with a federal law to back this change!"

"Martin Luther King had a dream," Dr. Atkins wrote. "I, too, have one."

"THE DIET FAD OF THE 21ST CENTURY"

Allowing a good 20 years for dieters to forget, the book was reissued as *Dr. Atkins' New Diet Revolution* in 1992 (though there was not much new about it). Revived along with VW bugs and other retro '70s fashions, and this time backed by an aggressive marketing campaign, it became the best-selling fad-diet book in history, achieving "fashion-cult status amongst society figures."

What may have truly made it "the diet fad of the 21st century" (as an editor of the *Journal of the American Dietetics Association* dubbed it) came a decade later with the publication of the infamous pro-Atkins *New York Times Magazine* article "What if it's all been a big fat lie?" Atkins quickly wrote an editorial for his website claiming the article "validated" his work. Gushingly favorable follow-up stories appeared on NBC's *Dateline*, CBS' *48 Hours*, and ABC's *20/20*. The Atkins Corporation claimed literally billions of media hits. By the time the article's many flaws were exposed weeks later, the book had already catapulted to #1 on the *New York Times* paperback bestseller list. Atkins' net worth zoomed to $100 million.

The piece was written by freelance writer and Atkins advocate Gary Taubes (who reportedly scored a book deal from it—and a $700,000 advance). When the *Washington Post* investigated his pro-Atkins article, they found that Taubes simply ignored all the research that didn't agree with his conclusions.

Taubes evidently interviewed a number of prominent obesity researchers and then twisted their words. "What frightens me," said Barbara Rolls, an obesity expert at Pennsylvania State University, "is that he picks and chooses his facts. . . . If the facts don't fit in with his yarn, he ignores them."

The article seemed to claim that experts recommended the

diet. "I was greatly offended at how Gary Taubes tricked us all into coming across as supporters of the Atkins Diet," said John Farquhar, a Professor Emeritus of Medicine at Stanford. When the director of the Center for Human Nutrition at the Washington University School of Medicine was asked to comment on one of Taubes' claims, he replied, "It's preposterous."

"The article was written in bad faith," said F. Xavier Pi-Sunyer, director of the Obesity Research Center at St. Luke's-Roosevelt Hospital Center in New York. "It was irresponsible." "I think he's a dangerous man," said Farquhar, "I'm sorry I ever talked to him." Referring to the book deal, "Taubes sold out."

What the researchers stressed was how dangerous saturated fat and meat consumption could be, but Taubes seemed to have conveniently left it all out. "The article was incredibly misleading," said the pioneering Stanford University endocrinologist Gerald Reaven. "I ended up being embarrassed as hell. He sort of set me up. . . . I was horrified."

THE SOUTH BEACH DIET: ALL WET

The majority of the best-selling diet titles in history have been sold just during the last five years. One of the latest "steak oil" salesmen is Dr. Arthur Agatston, whose *South Beach Diet* appeared a year after Atkins' latest and sold its first million copies in just two months. Within months of publication, subscriptions to his website alone reportedly brought in a million dollars a week.

The *Tufts University Health and Nutrition Letter* weighed in on the South Beach Diet in its May 2004 issue: "Disappointingly, the South Beach Diet is simply yet another version of a fad wrapped within a gimmick." The authors concluded that the diet was "based on fallacies . . . replete with faulty science, glaring nutritional inaccuracies, contradictions, and claims of scientific evidence minus the actual evidence."

The article notes, "The faulty and confusing science is compounded by the South Beach Diet's own internal inconsistencies." The *Harvard Health Letter*, for example, noted that, while Agatston claims up front that his diet doesn't depend on exercise, he later tells people to get 20 minutes a day. In Phase II, he first tells readers to avoid bananas, then goes on to recommend bananas dipped in chocolate sauce. He claims at first that the diet is "distinguished by the absence of calorie counting or even rules about portion size" and that one shouldn't "even think about limiting the amount you eat." However, Agatston counts calories and measures out servings every step of the way, even to the point of specifying "I recommend counting out 15 almonds or cashews." That sounded like a rule about portion size to the reviewers.

Tufts lists a few of the "out-and-out food and nutrition inaccuracies" in *The South Beach Diet*. Agatston says that whole wheat bread is not whole-grain, but cous cous is (actually, the reverse is true). He claims watermelon is full of sugar but cantaloupe is not (they have the same amount). He claims eggs have minimal saturated fat—wrong. Each egg can have as much as 2 grams, giving some of his recipes over a third of one's daily limit. For a cardiologist who claims, "I feel nearly as comfortable in the world of nutrition as I do among cardiologists," Dr. Agatston "sprinkled an awful lot of nutrition gaffes throughout his book," the Tufts letter stated.

To be fair, he does frown on lard, although the Atkins Corporation is quick to point out that the South Beach menus do not have significantly less saturated fat than Atkins. Indeed, just as Dr. Atkins claimed he followed his diet for decades but was overweight according to his own cardiologist, Agatston revealed that he needs to take medication to lower his cholesterol.

THE LOW-CARB LOWDOWN

Though we've seen that every low-carb diet fad eventually falls out of favor, each in its time ends up endangering the health of millions of Americans. Shortly after Atkins' original book was published, the highly prestigious *Medical Letter on Drugs and Therapeutics* concluded that the Atkins Diet was "unbalanced, unsound and unsafe." A *Medical Times* review noted that Atkins had created a "ridiculously unbalanced and unsound," "hazardous" diet. Twenty-seven years later the *Medical Letter* offered an update noting that the safety of the Atkins Diet had still "not been established."

This is hardly surprising when we consider that recent medical reviews have called Atkins' feel-good theories "factually flawed" and "at best half-truths." "In the scientific world, books like *The Zone Diet* are generally regarded as fiction," one reviewer wrote in the *Journal of the American College of Nutrition*. "The scientific literature is in opposition. . . ." In a medical journal article entitled "Food—fads and fallacies," the Atkins Diet is referred to as a "new wives' tale" with a "sprinkling of fallacies." In an article entitled "Americans love hogwash," Edward H. Rynearson, Emeritus Professor of Medicine at the Mayo Clinic, singled out Dr. Atkins for his "worthless, false or ridiculous speech or writings" and praised the American Medical Association for "condemning this diet for its dangers." The "evidence" cited by Atkins has been called "nearly all anecdotal and misleading."

Indeed, a 2003 review of low-carb "theories" in the *Journal of the American College of Nutrition* concluded: "When properly evaluated, the theories and arguments of popular low-carbohydrate diet books . . . rely on poorly controlled, non-peer-reviewed studies, anecdotes and non-science rhetoric. . . . A closer look at the science behind the claims made for [these books] reveals nothing more than a modern twist on an antique food fad." We'll take that closer look in the next chapter.

CHAPTER 2

FAULTY SCIENCE

....

PHONY BALONEY

ONE OF DR. ATKINS' DREAMS PROBABLY CAME TRUE—HE LIKELY became a billionaire before he died. Backed by multi-billion-dollar investment bankers like Goldman Sachs and Company, the Atkins empire (though it doesn't like to "talk about its profits") was estimated by *Fortune* magazine in 2004 to be worth over two billion dollars. However, as one doctor put it in *Family Practice News*, "Unfortunately, Dr. Robert C. Atkins, who made a lot of money playing on the ignorance of Americans, knew about as much about nutrition as an Arkansas hog knows about astronomy." Is it too much to ask that cardiologists like Dr. Atkins know something about nutrition?

The entire theoretical framework of low-carb diets, like Atkins and The Zone, hangs upon the notion that insulin, a hormone that facilitates fat storage, is the root of all evil. To limit insulin release, low-carb diet gurus state, one needs to limit carbohydrate intake. Dr. Atkins, for example, has a chapter entitled "Insulin—The Hormone That Makes You Fat." *Protein Power* calls it the "monster hormone," and the author of *The Zone Diet* calls insulin "the single most significant determinant of your weight."

What they overlook is that "protein- and fat-rich foods may induce substantial insulin secretion" as well, according to the *American Journal of Clinical Nutrition*. Research in which study subjects served as their own controls, for example, has shown that under fasting conditions a quarter pound of beef raises insulin levels in diabetics as much as a quarter pound of straight sugar.

Featured foods of the Atkins Diet include cheese and beef, which elevate insulin levels higher than "dreaded" high-carbohydrate foods like pasta. A single burger's worth of beef, or three slices of cheddar cheese, boosts insulin levels more than almost 2 cups of cooked pasta. In fact a study in the *American Journal of Clinical Nutrition* found that when blood-sugar releases were examined, meat seems to cause the most insulin secretion of any food tested.

Low-carb advocates like Atkins seem to completely ignore these facts. According to a 2003 article in the *Journal of the American Medical Association*, "Dr. Atkins and his colleagues selectively recite the literature" to support their claims.

A study done at Tufts, for example, presented at the 2003 American Heart Association convention, compared four popular diets for a year: Weight Watchers, the Zone Diet, the Atkins Diet (almost no carbs), and the Ornish Diet (almost all carbs). The insulin levels of those instructed to go on the Ornish diet dropped 27%. Out of the four diets that were compared that year, Ornish's vegetarian diet was the only one to significantly lower the "monster hormone" that "makes you fat," even though that's supposedly what the Atkins and the Zone diets were designed to do.

In another study, researchers took over a hundred pairs of identical twins and found that the more fat they ate, the *higher* their resting insulin levels became. Even with the same genes, when one twin ate more fat and less carbs, the study "showed a consistent pattern of higher fasting insulin levels with intake of high-fat, low-carbohydrate diets."

Other studies show that a diet high in carbohydrates (70–85%), combined with a 15- to 30-minute walk a day, can result not only in significant reductions in body weight, blood pressure, cholesterol, and triglycerides, but significant drops in baseline insulin levels as well—exactly the opposite of what low-carb pushers would predict. In just three weeks on a vegetarian diet high in unrefined carbohydrates, along with a few minutes of daily walking, diabetics reduced the amount of insulin they needed, and most of those identified as pre-diabetics seemed cured of their insulin resistance. In general, vegetarians may have half the insulin levels of nonvegetarians, even at the same weight.

LOSING (WATER) WEIGHT

The director of Yale University's Center for Eating and Weight Disorders details the miracle formula used by diet books to become bestsellers for over a century now: "easy, rapid weight loss; the opportunity to eat your favorite foods and some scientific 'breakthrough' that usually doesn't exist."

We know that the Atkins Diet is successful—at making money. But how does it fare when it comes to weight loss? We know that cutting down on carbs will help people lose variety and nutrition in their diet—and if they buy the Atkins-recommended supplements, their wallets may get slimmer—but what about their waistlines?

Who cares if the American Medical Association calls Atkins' theory "naive," "biochemically incorrect," "inaccurate," and "without scientific merit"? Who cares if it "doesn't make physiological sense"? The question is, does it work?

Carbohydrates burn cleanly. In fact, the name "carbohydrate" basically means "carbon (dioxide) and water," which are what plants make carbs out of. Carbon dioxide and water, for that matter, is all the waste product one is left with when the body uses carbohydrates as fuel. During the first few weeks of the Atkins Diet, the so-called "induction" phase, a person is forced to live off so much grease that, lacking the preferred fuel—carbohydrates—the body goes into starvation mode.

In biochemistry class, doctors learn that fat "burns in the flame of carbohydrate." When one is eating enough carbohydrates, fat can be completely broken down as well. But when one's body runs out of carb fuel to burn, its only choice is to burn fat inefficiently using a pathway that produces toxic byproducts like acetone and other so-called "ketones." The acetone escapes through the lungs—giving Atkins followers what one weight-loss expert calls "rotten-apple breath"—and the other ketones have to be excreted by the kidneys. We burn fat all the time; it's only when we are carbohydrate-deficient and have to burn fat inefficiently that we go into what's called a state of ketosis, defined as having so much acetone in our blood that it noticeably spills out into our lungs, or so many other ketones that they spill out into our urine.

To wash these toxic waste products out of our system, the body uses a lot of water. The diuretic effect of low-carb diets can result in people losing a gallon of water in pounds the first week. This precipitous early weight loss encourages dieters to continue the diet even though they have lost mostly water weight and the state of ketosis may be making them nauseated or worse. If one wanted to try to lose water weight, sweating it away in a sauna might be a more healthful way.

The initial rapid loss of water weight that is typically seen on low-carb diets has an additional sales benefit. By the time people gain back the weight, they may have already told all their friends to buy the book. This, says the *Journal of the American Medical Association*, explains why low-carb diets have been such "cash cows" for publishers over the last 140 years. As one weight-loss expert notes, "Rapid water loss is the $33-billion diet gimmick."

CALORIES COUNT

When people do lose weight on the Atkins Diet after the first few weeks, it's almost certainly because they are eating fewer calories. People lose weight on the Atkins Diet the same way they lost weight on the 1941 Grapefruit Diet, the 1963 Hot Dog Diet, the 2002 Ice Cream Diet, and every other fad diet promising a quick fix—by restricting calories.

In 2001, the medical journal *Obesity Research* published "Popular diets: A scientific review." Claiming to have reviewed every study ever done on low-carb diets, they concluded, "In all cases, individuals on high-fat, low-carbohydrate diets lose weight because they consume fewer calories." Calories count—every time, all the time. "No magic ingredients, strange food combinations or pseudoscientific formulas will alter this metabolic fact."

Dr. Atkins disagreed. In fact, he accused his critics of having "subnormal intellects" for even holding such a view. For three decades he peddled his claim that people could eat more calories and still lose weight. Decrying what he called the "calorie hoax," Atkins had a chapter entitled "How to Stay Fat—Keep Counting Calories." Atkins even subtitled his book "The High Calorie Way to Stay Thin Forever." *The Zone Diet* made a similar claim on its back cover: "You can burn more fat by watching TV than by exercising." (As one commentator exclaimed, "Goodness, what channel does he watch?")

Atkins claimed people could lose 85 pounds, without exercising, eating an incredible 5,500 calories a day. The only problem, critics claimed, was that this ran counter to the first law of thermodynamics, considered to be the most fundamental law in the universe. No wonder the AMA scolded Atkins' publishers for promoting "bizarre concepts of nutrition and dieting."

"METABOLIC ADVANTAGE" ADVANTAGEOUS
ONLY IN SELLING BOOKS

Atkins claimed that dieters in ketosis urinate and breathe out so many calories in the form of ketones that "weight will be lost even when the calories taken in far exceed the calories expended." He claimed dieters could "sneak" calories out of the body unused.

The "Atkins Physicians Council" also claims that one's body expends more energy burning fat and thus "You wouldn't have to increase your exercise at all because your body would be working harder, so that you could literally sit in your armchair and lose weight." In the words of the secretary of the AMA's Council on Food and Nutrition, "The whole [Atkins] diet is so replete with errors woven together that it makes the regimen sound mysterious and magical."

These claims sounded so far-fetched that, as part of an investigative documentary, the BBC paid obesity researchers to design an experiment to test it. So researchers took two identical twins and put one on the Atkins Diet for a while, the other on a high-carbohydrate diet. They locked them both in sealed chambers to measure exactly where the calories were going. Did the twin on the Atkins Diet have any metabolic "advantage" by burning fat and protein as his source of fuel? Was he literally flushing more calories down the toilet? Of course not. "We found no difference [in calories burned] whatsoever," the researcher said.

As the evidently "subnormal intellects" at the AMA concluded, "No scientific evidence exists to suggest that the low-carbohydrate ketogenic diet has a metabolic advantage over more conventional diets for weight reduction." The only comprehensive systematic review ever done of low-carb diets found that neither the carbohydrate nor the protein content of one's diet is in any way particularly correlated with weight loss. Ultimately, the truth seems to be that nothing matters more than calories when it comes to weight loss. According to the director of nutrition at the Center for Science in the Public Interest, "This whole ketosis thing is just a gimmick to make people think there's something to blame for weight gain and some magic solution to take it off. That's the beginning and end of it."

But what about all the scientific studies Dr. Atkins cited in his book to back up his claims? Although his first book had essentially no citations, by the final edition he listed over 300. Reviewing all of the studies on low-carb diets, researchers concluded, "The studies by Atkins to support his contentions were of limited duration, conducted on a small number of people, lacked adequate controls and used ill-defined diets." Most importantly, though, some of the very studies he cites actually *refute* the claims he's making.

Of the few studies that do back up his claims, some have seriously questionable validity, and researchers could not replicate the findings of the rest. One review of studies that have defended Atkins claims concluded, "It turns out that when these data are critically analyzed they are often found to be in error, and it's therefore impossible to accept the validity of the conclusions derived by the authors from such erroneous data."

LOW-CALORIE DIET IN DISGUISE

The Atkins Diet restricts calories by restricting choices. If all one did was eat Twinkies, one could lose weight (unless one were able to consistently force oneself to eat more than a dozen a day). But would one's overall health be the better for it?

Americans get half of their energy from carbohydrates, so if they cut out half the food they eat, what they are left with is calorie restriction. Yes, one can eat unlimited amounts of fat on the Atkins Diet, but people typically can't stomach an extra two sticks of butter's worth a day to make up for the calorie deficit. Since so many foods are taboo, people end up eating less out of sheer boredom and lack of variety. As one obesity researcher put it, "If you're only allowed to shop in two aisles of the grocery store, does it matter which two they are?"

Yes, all the butter one can eat, but no bread to put it on. All the cream cheese, but no bagels. Sour cream, but no baked potato. Lunch meat, but no sandwiches. Cheese, but no mac. Having all the mayonnaise one can eat only goes so far. Atkins told readers of *Australian Magazine* how to make cheeseburgers without the bun: "I put all the meat on the outside . . . put the cheese on the inside. . . . The cheese melts on the inside and never gets out." Although his recipe for "hamburger fondue," combining burger meat, blue cheese, and butter, may top the cheeseburger recipe for heart disease risk, first prize would probably go to his recipe for "Swiss Snack," which consists of wrapping bacon strips around cubes of Swiss cheese and deep frying them in hot oil. The recipe, which supposedly serves one, calls for four strips of bacon and a quarter-pound of cheese.

And then there are pork rinds. Described as the "secret manna of every Atkins dieter," pork rinds are chunks of pigs' skin that are deep-fried, salted and artificially flavored. Atkins recommends that people use them to dip caviar. Or, perhaps for those who can't afford caviar, one can use fried pork rinds as a "substitute for toast, dinner rolls. . . . You can use them as a pie crust . . . or even matzo ball soup (see our recipe on p. 190)." Matzo balls made out of pork rinds?—now that *is* a diet revolution!

THE *REAL* BIG FAT LIE

In his article in the *New York Times Magazine*, Gary Taubes reiterated a myth common among proponents of greasy diets: "At the very moment that the government started telling Americans to eat less fat, we got fatter." He argues that since the percentage of calories from fat in the American diet has been decreasing, and the percentage from carbohydrates increasing, carbs are to blame for the obesity epidemic.

Of course, a quick trot across the globe shows that some of the thinnest populations in the world, like those in rural Asia, center their entire diets on carbs. They eat 50% more carbs than we do, yet have a fraction of our obesity rates. Taubes also left out that, though the *percentage* of fat in the American diet has decreased, the *amount* of fat we eat has actually been increasing—we're eating more of everything now, fat *and* carbohydrates. Grease and protein peddlers blame our obesity epidemic on low-fat diets that no one really adheres to.

Thirty years ago, the average woman ate about 1,500 calories per day; now it's closer to 2,000. Men have also significantly bumped up their calorie consumption. With that many extra calories, we'd have to walk about two extra hours a day to keep from gaining weight. As analyzed in the May 2004 USDA report on obesity, adding those calories without altering our sedentary lifestyle guaranteed we'd gain weight.

Bread and fruit are not the culprits here. Much of the obesity crisis has been blamed on eating out more (Americans spend almost twice as much time per week eating out as exercising), soft drinks, snacking, and bigger portion sizes. Twenty years ago, a typical U.S. bagel was 3 inches in diameter; now it's twice that and contains a whopping 350 calories. One steakhouse has an appetizer of cheese fries that breaks the scale at over 3,000 calories, more calories than most people eat all day. One would have to walk about 35 miles to burn that kind of thing off.

The standard Coke bottle used to be around 6 ounces. Then came the 12-ounce can. Now we have 20-ounce bottles and the 64-ounce "Double Gulp," containing about 50 spoonfuls of sugar. In fact, the Double Gulp is selling so well that 7-Eleven considered an even larger size, which a company spokesperson described only as a "wading-pool-sized drink."

The National Soft Drink Association boasts on its website that "Soft drinks have emerged as America's favorite refreshment. Indeed, one of every four beverages consumed in America today is a carbonated soft drink, averaging out to about 52 gallons of soft drinks per year for every man, woman and child." Interestingly, the introduction of high-fructose corn syrup (primarily consumed in soft drinks) around 1970 seems to exactly parallel the sudden rapid rise in obesity in this country.

In the medical literature, the obesity epidemic has been blamed in part on "the enormous amount of very clever and very effective advertising of junk food/fast food." Coca-Cola alone, for example, spends up to $2 billion a year on advertising. Our children are subjected to 10,000 ads for processed food every year. There's no way parents can compete. As another medical journal pointed out, our children "will never see a slick high-budget (or even low-budget) ad for apples or broccoli." Thanks in part to American food corporations, becoming overweight, as one prominent obesity researcher pointed out, "is now the normal response to the American environment."

It's no mystery why we are the fattest country on Earth. "We're overfed, over-advertised, and under-exercised," says Stanford obesity expert John Farquhar. "It's the enormous portion sizes and sitting in front of the TV and computer all day" that are to blame. "It's so gol' darn obvious—how can anyone ignore it?"

CHAPTER 3

ALL LONG-TERM STUDIES ON ATKINS A WASH

·····················

ATKINS COMES IN LAST FOR LONG-TERM WEIGHT MAINTENANCE

SO FINE, MAYBE CALORIES, NOT CARBOHYDRATES, ARE TO BLAME for our obesity epidemic, and maybe Atkins' claims, as described by one of the world's leading obesity researchers, are "the most unutterable nonsense I ever saw in my life." So what if it's just a low-calorie diet in disguise? It's still a low-calorie diet where you can eat all the (albeit bunless) bacon cheeseburgers you want. So what's the problem?

Anyone can lose weight on a diet; the critical question is whether the weight loss can be maintained and at what cost. If low-carb diets really did cure obesity, the original in 1864 would have eliminated the problem and no more diet revolutions would be necessary.

The problem with low-carb diets is that short-term weight loss is not the same thing as lifelong weight maintenance—and there are no data to show that the initial rapid weight loss on the Atkins Diet can be maintained long term. Many of the studies on the Atkins Diet have lasted only a few days; the longest the Atkins Diet has been formally studied and reported to date is one year.

There have been four such yearlong studies, and not a single one showed significantly more weight lost at the end of the year with the Atkins Diet than with the control diets. In the yearlong study that compared the Atkins Diet to Ornish's diet, Weight Watchers, and the Zone Diet, the Atkins Diet came in dead *last* in terms of weight loss. By the end of the year, half of the Atkins group had dropped out, and those who remained ended up an unimpressive 4% lighter. Ornish's vegetarian diet seemed to show the most weight loss. The Atkins website had no comment.

Ornish's vegetarian (near-vegan) diet has been formally tested for years. Even though the diet was not even designed for weight loss, after five years most of the Ornish adherents were able to maintain much of the first year's 24-pound weight loss "even though they were eating more food, more frequently, than before without hunger or deprivation."

Another of the yearlong studies compared a low-fat vegan diet* to the Atkins Diet. Results showed that those who ate as much as they wanted on the vegan diet lost a whopping 52 pounds on average—60% more than the average weight loss of those reportedly on the Atkins Diet. This is consistent with what research we have on vegans themselves.

The biggest study on vegans to date compared over 1,000 vegans in Europe to tens of thousands of meat eaters and vegetarians. The meat eaters, on average, were significantly heavier than the vegetarians, who were in turn significantly heavier than the vegans. Even after controlling for exercise, smoking, and other nondietary factors, vegans came out slimmest in every age

---

*Vegans are vegetarians who exclude all saturated animal fat and cholesterol from their diet.

group. Less than 2% of vegans were obese, compared to almost a third of the American public.

In a snapshot of the diets of 10,000 Americans, vegetarians were the slimmest, whereas those eating the fewest carbs in the sample weighed the most. Those eating fewer carbs were on average overweight; those eating vegetarian were not.

Vegetarians may have a higher resting metabolic rate, which researchers chalk up to their eating more carbs than meat eaters do (or possibly to enhanced adrenal function). At the same weight, one study showed that vegetarians seem to burn more calories per minute just by sitting around or sleeping than meat eaters—almost 200 extra calories a day. Although earlier studies didn't find such an effect, if confirmed, that amounts to the equivalent of an extra pound of fat a month burned off by choosing to eat vegetarian.

The other two formal yearlong studies found that although the initial drop in weight on the Atkins Diet was more rapid, the weight loss reversed or stalled after six months. The longer people stayed on the Atkins Diet, the worse they seemed to do, and none of the three longest studies of the Atkins Diet showed any significant advantage over those types of high-carbohydrate diets Atkins blamed for making America fat.

LONG-TERM WEIGHT LOSS SECRETS

Permanent weight control is difficult to achieve. Up to approximately 95% of repeat dieters fail, regaining the weight that they initially lost. In her book *Eating Thin for Life*, award-winning journalist and dietician Anne Fletcher delved into the habits of a few hundred representatives of the other 5%—folks who had not only lost an average of 64 pounds but also maintained that loss for an average of 11 years. What did she find?

"[B]asically, they're eating the opposite of a high-protein, low-carbohydrate diet," Fletcher reported. When she asked them to describe their eating habits, the top responses were "low fat" followed by "eating less meat."

These dieters with long-term success also told her they ate "more fruits and vegetables." Research seems to support this notion. One research study showed, for example, that significant weight loss could be triggered in people just by feeding them extra fruit—three added apples or pears a day. The results of a Harvard study of 75,000 women over a decade suggest that the more fruits and vegetables women eat, the less likely they are to become obese. A 2004 review of the available research suggests that in general "increasing fruit and vegetable intake may be an important strategy for weight loss."

Researchers at the National Cancer Institute followed over 75,000 people for 10 years to find out which behaviors were most associated with weight loss and which with weight gain. They wrapped tape measures around people's waists for a decade and found that the one dietary behavior most associated with an expanding waistline was high meat consumption. And the dietary behavior most strongly associated with a loss of abdominal fat was high vegetable consumption.

Even after controlling for other factors, men and women who ate more than a single serving of meat per day seemed to be 50% more likely to suffer an increase in abdominal obesity than those who ate meat just a few times per week. The researchers conclude: "Our analysis has identified several easily described behaviors [such as reducing meat intake to less than three servings per week and jogging a few hours every week] that, if widely adopted, might help reverse recent increases in adult overweight. . . . Increases in vegetable consumption might reduce abdominal obesity even further."

The sad thing, according to the director of nutrition for the Center for Science in the Public Interest, is that "people keep believing that the magic bullet is just around the corner . . . if they only eliminate food 'x' or combine foods 'a' and 'b,' or twirl around three times before each meal." The reality is that most successful dieters lose weight without the gimmicks on which Americans spend $30 billion per year.

A recent survey of 1,300 adults found that low-carb diets seemed to be 50% less effective in helping people reach their weight-loss goals than weight-loss diets in general. In the largest survey undertaken to date on the long-term maintenance of weight loss, *Consumer Reports* found that the vast majority of the most successful dieters said they lost weight entirely on their own, without enrolling in any program, or buying special foods or supplements, or following the regimen of some diet guru. Atkins may be the most popular *fad* diet right now, but it's not the most popular diet, or the one that seems to work the best.

ATKINS MISSING IN ACTION

The most formal study of lasting weight loss is the highly respected National Weight Control Registry, funded by the National Institutes of Health. For over 10 years, the Registry has tracked the habits of thousands of successful dieters. They now have 5,000 Americans confirmed to have lost an average of 70 pounds (32 kg), who were able to keep it off for an average of six years. After a decade of rigorously tracking those who most successfully lost weight—and kept it off—one of the chief investigators revealed what they found: "Almost nobody's on a low-carbohydrate diet."

These researchers, led by a team at Brown University and the University of Colorado, found that the people most successful in losing and maintaining their weight were eating *high*-carbohydrate diets—five times as many carbs as Atkins prescribed in the "weight loss" phase of his diet. Of the thousands of people in the National Weight Control Registry, less than 1% follow a diet similar to the Atkins program. "We can't find more than a handful of people who follow the Atkins program in the registry," said one chief investigator, "and, believe me, we've tried."

Fifteen million Atkins books sold and investigators can only find a "handful" of followers who could qualify for the Registry? To qualify, all dieters have to do is prove they lost just 30 pounds and kept it off for at least one year. Twenty-six million Americans supposedly on "hard-core" low-carb diets and "almost nobody" on Atkins has even qualified?

Maybe for some reason only dieters eating lots of carbohydrates hear about the Registry? No, the National Weight Control Registry has been plugged in Dr. Atkins' own book for years and is promoted on the official Atkins website. The reason anecdotes of Atkins dieters maintaining their weight loss crop up in Atkins books and websites, but seemingly nowhere else, may be that there isn't much oversight when posting information to the web, whereas the Registry demands proof.

BRINGING HOME THE BACON

Atkins conceded that the "WORST" (emphasis his) feature about his diet is the "rapidity with which you gain [weight] if you abandon it. . . . But the BEST feature," he claims, "is that you don't HAVE to go off this diet. . . ."

The reason people fall off the wagon, Atkins claimed, is "carbohydrate addiction." What he calls "addiction," though, others might call our natural urge to eat the fuel our bodies evolved to live on—carbohydrates. Patients inevitably cheat and then blame themselves instead of the diet for this failure.

Low-carb diets, like all fad diets, tend to fail. Even Atkins admitted that there is "no formal documentation" of long-term weight loss on his diet. He'd supposedly been seeing patients for decades on his diet; why didn't he do a study? When challenged on that point, Atkins replied, "Why should I support a study? It's all in my book." When it was pointed out that the book was "all anecdotal," Atkins said mainstream medicine's demand for proof simply functioned to "maintain it at its current level of ineptitude."

In February 2000, the USDA brought Atkins in to discuss his diet. When asked why he didn't conduct his own study, he pleaded poverty: "But I haven't been able to fund a study." To which the director of nutrition sciences at Albert Einstein College of Medicine replied, "Ten million books in print and you can't fund a study?" The director continued: "You market the vitamins. You sell the vitamins. You market this. This is not for the public good. This is a money-making proposition." The chair of the board of Atkins' own New York County Medical Society made a similar charge when Atkins' book was first published, alleging it was "clearly . . . unethical" and "self-aggrandizing." The New York Board of Health later tried, unsuccessfully, to revoke Atkins' medical license.

Why has the U.S. government been lax in testing the Atkins Diet at any point in the last 30 years? Perhaps it's difficult to get approval from an ethical review committee, since the long-term dangers of a meat-laden diet are unknown. As one medical review concluded, "There is no evidence that low-carbohydrate diets are effective for long-term weight management, and their long-term safety is questionable and unproven." Even in the short term, Atkins dieters risk an array of side effects that range from unpleasant all the way to life-threatening, as we are about to see.

CHAPTER 4

SHORT-TERM SIDE EFFECTS

....

"EXTRAORDINARILY IRRESPONSIBLE"
—ATKINS AND PREGNANCY

The immediate concern regarding the Atkins Diet centers on the state of ketosis, which occurs during the induction phase. Pregnant women are the most at risk. Based on detailed data from 55,000 pregnancies, acetone and other ketones in the bloodstream may cause brain damage in the fetus, which may result in the baby being born mentally retarded. The fact that ketones seemed to cause "significant neurological impairment" and an average loss of about 10 IQ points was well known and aroused "considerable concern" years before Atkins published his first book. Atkins nonetheless wrote, "I recommend this diet to all my pregnant patients."

After enough pressure from the American Medical Association, Atkins finally relented, admitting: "I now understand that ketosis during pregnancy could result in fetal damage. . . . My pregnant patients have never had this problem, but I realize I didn't study enough cases to validate my recommendation. If anyone wants a retraction, I'll be glad to give one."

Subsequently, however, when asked by Senator George McGovern at the congressional hearing on fad diets if he had made a public retraction of his reckless recommendation, Atkins replied, "No; I will stand by the statement I made in the book. . . . I have recommended it for use by the pregnant woman with the observation of the managing obstetrician or physician. . . ." Just the same, after the Senate Select Committee hearings, Atkins' publisher added a small-print disclaimer to the copyright page in the front of the book.

Highlighting Atkins' recommendation of his diet even during pregnancy, one nutrition textbook reads, "Proponents of the low-carbohydrate diet have been extraordinarily irresponsible in ignoring these hazards." The tobacco industry similarly denied that smoking was harmful during pregnancy. "The woman who goes on a ketogenic diet [like Atkins'] for six months of pregnancy," noted one fetal specialist, "is playing Russian roulette."

MORE TO LOSE THAN WEIGHT

Although pregnant and breastfeeding women may be most at risk, "The [Atkins] diet is potentially dangerous to everyone," warned the chair of the Medical Society of New York County's Public Health Committee. In all of the editions of his *Diet Revolution*, Atkins cited the "pioneering" work of "brilliant" researcher Gaston Pawan. When Atkins was brought before the Senate investigation on fad diets, however, the chair of the Senate Subcommittee read a statement submitted by Dr. Pawan himself supporting the AMA's condemnation of the Atkins Diet. Dr. Pawan's statement explained that he used very high-fat diets only for "specific *experimental* purposes" (emphasis in original) in hospital settings and would never "recommend a very high-fat diet indiscriminately to obese subjects for obvious reasons."

The symptoms of ketosis include general tiredness, abrupt or gradually increasing weakness, dizziness, headaches, confusion,

abdominal pain, irritability, nausea and vomiting, sleep problems, and bad breath. One study found that all those subjected to
carb-free diets complained of fatigue after just two days. "[T]his
complaint was characterized by a feeling of physical lack of
energy. . . . The subjects all felt that they did not have sufficient
energy to continue normal activity after the third day. This
fatigue promptly disappeared after the addition of carbohydrates
to the diet." From a review published in a German medical journal, "[lightheadedness], fatigue, and nausea are frequent, despite
what Dr. Atkins claims."

In World War II, the Canadian Army had an illuminating
experience with ketogenic diets. For emergency rations, infantry
troops were compelled to eat pemmican, a carbohydrate-free
mixture of beef jerky and suet (animal fat). The performance of
the infantrymen forced to live on such a limited diet deteriorated
so rapidly that the troops were actually incapacitated in a matter
of days. As reported in the journal *War Medicine* in 1945, "On the
morning of the fourth day of the diet, physical examination
revealed a group of listless, dehydrated men with drawn faces
and sunken eyeballs, whose breath smelled strongly of acetone."
A ketogenic diet, concluded one medical review, "can be associated with significant toxicity."

Danish obesity expert Arne Astrup, M.D., of the Centre of
Advanced Food Research in Copenhagen, published a review of
the Atkins Diet in *The Lancet*, one of the most prestigious medical journals in the world, in September 2004. Long-term Atkins
adherents "start to suffer headaches, muscle cramps and diarrhea," Astrup concluded. "This is consistent with a carbohydrate
deficiency. They simply do not get enough carbohydrate to supply the tissues with blood sugar. That is why the organs start to
malfunction."

In a study funded by Atkins himself, most of the people who
could stick with the diet reported headaches and halitosis (bad

breath). Ten percent suffered hair loss. While most people lost weight—at least in the short-term—70% of the patients in the study also lost the ability to have a normal bowel movement.

CONSTIPATION

Authorities recommend Americans start roughing it—so to speak—with "at least 30–35 grams" of fiber a day "from foods, not from supplements." The initial phase of the Atkins Diet, which dieters may have to repeatedly return to, has as little as 2 grams of fiber per day—that's less than 7% of the minimum daily requirement recommended by the American College of Gastroenterology.

Atkins can't help but concede the health benefits associated with fiber, which is found, in his own words, in "vegetables, nuts and seeds, fruits, beans and whole unrefined grains." But "How," he then asks in the latest edition of his book, "can you get the benefits of fiber without the carbs contained in these foods? The answer is supplementation." He then goes on to basically recommend that all his followers start taking sugar-free Metamucil. What must Mother Nature have been thinking, putting all the fiber into such "poison" foods?

A May 2004 *Annals of Internal Medicine* study—misleadingly lauded in the press with headlines like "Scientists give thumbs up to Atkins Diet"—showed once again that most Atkins dieters suffer from headaches and constipation. They also experience significantly more diarrhea, general weakness, rashes, and muscle cramps—despite taking the 65 supplements that Atkins prescribes. One subject was so constipated that he had to seek medical attention. Another developed chest pain on the diet and was subsequently diagnosed with coronary heart disease. No wonder *Consumer Guide* rated the Atkins Diet zero out of four stars for being "outright dangerous" and the editor of the *Healthy Weight Journal* gave Atkins the dubious Slim Chance Award for "Worst Diet."

"DISEASE OF KINGS"

Because of the Henry VIII-style meat load in low-carb diets (European royalty was known for its gluttony in centuries past), essentially every single study of these diets that measured uric acid levels showed that they rose. In virtually every instance in which it's been studied over the last 50 years, uric acid itself has been tied to cardiovascular disease risk, and may be an independent risk factor by increasing free radical damage or making the blood more susceptible to clotting.

There is also concern that uric acid levels on a meat-centered diet might be forced so high that the acid could start crystallizing in one's joints, triggering gout, an excruciating arthritic condition. A March 2004 article published in the *New England Journal of Medicine* documented the effects of meat intake on gout risk. Harvard researchers followed almost 50,000 men for 12 years and found that "each additional daily serving of meat was associated with a 21% increase in the risk of gout." In fact, the Atkins Diet has been blamed directly for the rising incidence of this so-called "disease of kings." Well, Atkins did claim his diet is "fit for a prince or princess."

PRESCRIPTION FOR MUSCLE CRAMPS

The presence of muscle cramps, Atkins explained, "means you are losing too many electrolytes." As they excrete ketones, the kidneys may also flush out critical electrolytes like calcium, magnesium and potassium, which may result in muscle cramps or worse.

Atkins realized this potential danger and recommended that his followers take potassium supplements. In fact, some people lose so much potassium that they may need professional help. According to Atkins himself, sales of potassium supplements "of anywhere near the proper amount of potassium you may need are illegal over the counter; therefore you may need a doctor to write you the proper prescription." Even Barry Sears, the author of the flawed Zone Diet, recognizes the danger the Atkins Diet might present: "Any meal that you have to take potassium supplements, there's something wrong with that."

MENTAL AND EMOTIONAL IMPAIRMENT

Experts have long been concerned that ketosis might fog up people's thinking, but this wasn't formally tested until 1995. As reported in the *International Journal of Obesity* article "Cognitive effects of ketogenic weight-reducing diets," researchers randomized people to either a ketogenic or a nonketogenic weight-loss diet. Although both groups lost the same amount of weight, those on the ketogenic diet suffered a significant drop in cognitive performance. After one week in ketosis, higher-order mental processing and mental flexibility significantly worsened into what the researcher called a "modest neuropsychological impairment."

The Atkins Diet may impair emotional functioning as well. Researchers at MIT have stated that the Atkins Diet is likely to make many people—especially women—irritable and depressed. The director of MIT's distinguished Clinical Research Center measured the serotonin levels in the brains of 100 volunteers eating different diets. (Serotonin is a chemical messenger in the brain that regulates mood. In fact, the way antidepressants like Prozac are purported to work is by increasing brain levels of this neurotransmitter.) The MIT researchers found that the brain only seemed to make serotonin after a person ate carbohydrates. By starving the brain of this essential mood elevator, the researchers fear that the Atkins Diet may make people restless, irritable, or depressed. They noted that women, people under stress, and those taking antidepressants might be most at risk.

Based on the MIT serotonin research, Judith Wurtman, director of the Women's Health Program at the MIT Research Center, warns that filling up on fatty foods like bacon or cheese may make people tired, lethargic and apathetic. Eating a lot of fat, she stated, may "make you an emotional zombie."

"SUNSHINE AND SEX"

Atkins' remedy to counteract or cover up the toxic effects of his diet is a list of prescriptions. Constipation? No problem, he says, take a laxative.

Leg cramps? They are "probably due to a calcium deficiency," Atkins explained. "I treat it with calcium supplements and vitamins E and C. Sometimes magnesium and potassium have to be added."

What if uric acid goes up? Not an obstacle for Atkins, who wrote: "This rarely poses a problem because I routinely prescribe a drug to prevent uric acid formation . . . if it goes above the normal range after being on the diet." He fails to mention, however, that this drug, allopurinol, when taken as prescribed, can cause irreversible liver damage, life-threatening anemia, and, in rare cases, even death.

Breath that smells "like a cross between nail polish and over-ripe pineapple"? Great—that means it's "working at full efficiency." Just "carry around . . . one of those purse-sized aerosol mouth fresheners, and you can have sweet breath. . . ."

Despite the side effects of ketosis, Atkins' books encourage people to repeatedly test their urine for ketones to ensure that they remain in this unhealthy state. Atkins almost fetishized ketosis, describing it being "as delightful as sunshine and sex." One dieter replied, "I don't think Dr. Atkins [has] had much sex if he thinks that ketosis is better than sex. It's certainly not." Incidentally, those who go on the Atkins Diet in an attempt to attract others may find it counterproductive when a potential mate gets too close and finds a constipated, cognitively impaired "zombie" with bad breath.

The current director of nutrition at Harvard advises that all physicians should produce a handout warning about all of the adverse effects of the Atkins Diet. These include not only " . . . dizziness, headaches, confusion, nausea, fatigue, sleep problems, irritability, bad breath, and worsening of gout and kidney problems; osteoporosis, since a high ratio of animal to vegetable protein intake may increase bone loss and the risk of hip fracture in elderly women; a rise in blood pressure with age . . . and rapid falling blood pressure upon standing up (orthostatic hypotension), which can . . . put older patients at higher risk for falls" but, in the long term, increased risk of heart disease, cancer and stroke. Thankfully, the short-term side effects are often so unpleasant that people don't stick with the diet for long. This downfall is also the Atkins Diet's one saving grace—people may not be able to tolerate it for long enough to suffer the long-term consequences.

CHAPTER 5

LONG-TERM SIDE EFFECTS

······················

"MASSIVE HEALTH RISK"

THE CHAIR OF THE AMERICAN MEDICAL ASSOCIATION'S COUNCIL on Food and Nutrition testified before the Senate Committee in 1973 as to why the AMA felt it had to publish an official condemnation of the Atkins Diet: "A careful scientific appraisal was carried out by several council and staff members, aided by outside consultants. It became apparent that the [Atkins] diet as recommended poses a serious threat to health."

The American Heart Association states: "Individuals who follow these [low-carb] diets are . . . at risk for compromised vitamin and mineral intake, as well as potential cardiac, renal [kidney], bone, and liver abnormalities overall." Low-carb diets like the Atkins Diet may also hasten the onset of type 2 diabetes. A 2002 review of the safety of these diets highlighted an alarming list of potential problems: "Complications such as heart arrhythmias, cardiac contractile function impairment, sudden death, osteoporosis, kidney damage, increased cancer risk, impairment of physical activity, and lipid [cholesterol] abnormalities can all be linked to long-term restriction of carbohydrates in the diet." In short, concluded a September 2004 review in the *Lancet*, "low-carbohydrate diets cannot be recommended."

In Europe, hospitals have already started banning the Atkins Diet since the British government's Medical Research Council, backed up by the British Nutrition Foundation and the British Dietetic Association, condemned the diet as "negligent . . . nonsense and pseudo-science" that poses a "massive health risk."

An article published in the *Cleveland Clinic Journal of Medicine*, entitled "Physician's guide to popular low-carbohydrate weight-loss diets," noted that the Atkins Diet "can jeopardize health in a variety of ways." Let us count the ways.

MALNUTRITION

Atkins' followers risk a number of serious nutritional deficiencies. As a 2004 review in the *Journal of the American College of Cardiology* concluded, the Atkins Diet is so "seriously deficient" in nutrition that "there is real danger of malnutrition in the long term." In fact, some people have become so deficient on low-carb ketogenic diets that they almost went blind because their optic nerves started to degenerate.

When cutting calories, it's especially important to eat nutrient-dense diets, but the Atkins Diet presents a double whammy: it restricts the healthiest foods, like fruit, and unrestricts some of the unhealthiest, like meat. Low-carbohydrate diets like Atkins maximize the consumption of disease-promoting substances like the cholesterol, saturated fat, and industrial pollutants found in meat, yet restrict one's intake of fiber and literally thousands of antioxidants and phytochemicals found exclusively in the plant kingdom (such as carotenoids, lycopenes, bioflavenoids, phytic acid, indoles, isothiocyanates, etc.) that have "anti-aging, anti-cancer and anti-heart-disease properties."

Where does one get one's vitamins on the Atkins Diet? From the Atkins website, of course, on sale now for just over $640 a year. Add some antioxidants and the tab is up to $1,000. (That is, of course, in addition to the estimated $400-$1,400 one must spend each month on the pricey Atkins foods—meat and cheese—that diet followers are encouraged to purchase. Of course, one can always choose to live on hot dogs). A "proper Atkins Dieter," Atkins wrote, "follows the entire program, including the supplements"—of which Atkins prescribed no less than 65 to fill the nutritional gaps in his diet. In the most recent edition of his book, Atkins even includes a chapter entitled "Nutritional Supplements: Don't Even Think of Getting Along Without Them." Perhaps this is because his corporation sells them.

"Who needs orange juice," Atkins wrote, "when a Vitamin C tablet is so handy?" Oranges, of course, contain much more than vitamin C. As Sue Radd, a world leader on phytonutrient research, put it, "There's not one vitamin pill in the world that can give you everything you need." A review in the *Cleveland Clinic Journal of Medicine* agreed that the Atkins Diet is "deficient in nutrients that cannot be replaced by supplements and . . . excessive in nutrients that may increase the risk of mortality and chronic disease."

Responding to the criticism that the Atkins Diet was deficient in fruits and vegetables, Atkins-funded researchers responded that dieters could include a limited quantity of some vegetables "and even small amounts of fruit." Even during later, more liberal phases of the diet, though, Atkins warned readers that eating fruit will "always be somewhat risky." The Atkins researchers continued, "It would be prudent to take a multivitamin/mineral supplement." A low-carb diet is a low-nutrition diet.

CANCER

Atkins' followers also risk cancer. Studies at Harvard and elsewhere involving tens of thousands of women and men have shown that regular meat consumption may increase colon cancer risk as much as 300%. As one Harvard School of Public Health researcher noted, because of the meat content, two years on the Atkins Diet "could initiate a cancer. It could show up as a polyp in 7 years and as colon cancer in 10." Another Harvard study showed that women with the highest intake of animal fat seem to have over a 75% greater risk of developing breast cancer.

As far back as 1892, *Scientific American* noted that "Cancer is most frequent among those branches of the human race where carnivorous habits prevail." This is nothing new. What's the number one recommendation of the American Institute for Cancer Research? Plant-based diets. The number one recommendation of the World Cancer Research Fund? Plant-based diets. The number one recommendation of the National Cancer Institute, the World Health Organization, and the Food and Agriculture Organization of the United Nations? More fruits and vegetables. The number one recommendation of the American Cancer Society? More plants, less meat. In fact, the American Cancer Society has officially condemned diets high in animal grease, concluding that "a low-carb diet can be a high-risk option when it comes to health."

KIDNEY DAMAGE

Atkins followers also risk kidney damage. Though Atkins once wrote, "The diet is safe for people even if there is a mild kidney malfunction," we now know this to be false.

In a press release entitled "American Kidney Fund warns about impact of high-protein diets on kidney health," the fund's chair of medical affairs, Paul W. Crawford, M.D., wrote, "We have long suspected that high-protein weight-loss diets could have a negative impact on the kidneys, and now we have research to support our suspicions." Dr. Crawford is worried that the strain put on the kidneys by the body's attempts to flush out the byproducts of the extra protein could result in irreversible scarring.

Three months later, the newest edition of *Dr. Atkins' New Diet Revolution* was released, in which Dr. Atkins stated: "Too many people believe this untruth [that too much protein is bad for your kidneys] simply because it is repeated so often that even intelligent health professionals assume it must have been reported somewhere. But the fact is that it has never been reported anywhere. I have yet to see someone produce a study for me to review. . . ."

Although evidence that such diets could be risky for one's kidneys existed years before he made that statement, the definitive study was published a month before Atkins died. The Harvard Nurses' Health Study proved that high meat protein intake was associated with an accelerated decline in kidney function in women with mild kidney insufficiency. The problem is that millions of Americans—as many as one in four adults in the United States—seem to already have reduced kidney function, but may not know it, and would potentially be harmed by a diet high in animal protein. And the "excessive" amount of protein that furthered kidney damage in the women in the Nurses' Study is only about half of what one might expect to get on the Atkins Diet.

The American Academy of Family Physicians notes that high animal protein intake is also largely responsible for the high prevalence of kidney stones in the United States. Kidney stones can cause severe pain, urinary obstruction, and kidney damage. Plant protein does not seem to have a harmful effect. "If we were smart," says Dr. Theodore Steinman, a kidney specialist and senior physician at Beth Israel Deaconess Medical Center, "we would all be vegetarians."

High cholesterol, which may be exacerbated by the Atkins Diet, has also been linked to a worsening of kidney function in both diabetics and nondiabetics.

The American Kidney Fund's Dr. Crawford concluded, "Chronic kidney disease is not to be taken lightly, and there is no cure for kidney failure. The only treatments are kidney dialysis and kidney transplantation. This research shows that even in healthy athletes, kidney function was impacted and that ought to send a message to anyone who is on a high-protein weight-loss diet."

PEEING YOUR BONES DOWN THE TOILET

There is a particular concern that children who go on the Atkins Diet might suffer permanent physical and mental damage as a result of starving their bodies of critical nutrients. As one U.S. child nutrition specialist explained, "The effect can be to dull the mind, stunt growth, and soften bones. . . . I wouldn't want to risk it by putting my child on a low-carbohydrate diet."

The concern with bone health arises from the fact that muscle protein has a high sulfur content. When people eat too much meat protein, the sulfur forms acid within their bodies that must somehow be neutralized to maintain a proper internal pH balance. One way our bodies can buffer the sulfuric acid load caused by meat is with calcium borrowed from our bones. Cheese is also a leading source of these sulfur-containing proteins. People on high-animal-protein diets can lose so much calcium in their urine that it can actually solidify into kidney stones. Over time, high animal protein intake may leach enough calcium from the bones to increase the risk of osteoporosis. Ultimately, people may be peeing their bones into the toilet along with the ketones.

The Harvard Nurses' Health Study, which followed over 85,000 nurses for a dozen years, found that those who ate more animal protein had a significantly higher risk of forearm fracture. While plant-based proteins did not show a deleterious effect, women eating just a serving of red meat a day seemed to have significantly increased fracture risk. Other studies have linked meat consumption to hip fracture risk as well.

Although Atkins conceded that "kidney stones are a conceivable complication," he dismissed any assertion that his diet might endanger bone health. Researchers decided to test his claim directly.

In 2002, researchers from the University of Chicago and the University of Texas published a study that put people on the Atkins Diet and measured both how acidic their urine got and just how much calcium was lost when they urinated. They reported that the Atkins Diet resulted in a "striking increase in net acid excretion." After just two weeks on the Atkins Diet, the subjects were already losing 258 mg of calcium in their urine every day. They concluded that the Atkins Diet "provides an exaggerated acid load, increasing risks for renal calculi [kidney stone] formation and bone loss." In addition, the Atkins Diet is actually deficient in calcium in the first place—even if one includes Atkins' recommended 65 supplements. Luckily there's a 66th, available on his website.

"EATERS OF RAW FLESH"

We don't have any long-term published data on the bone health of Atkins followers (or any other health parameter, for that matter). One might look to the Inuit peoples—the so-called "Eskimos"—for hints, though. (The word Eskimo comes from the word Eskimaux—"eaters of raw flesh.") They seem to be the only population on Earth approximating the Atkins Diet, living largely off Atkins' dream foods like blubber.

Despite having some of the highest calcium intakes in the world, the Inuit also have some of the worst rates of osteoporosis. Although calcium intakes vary widely, people in some villages get over 2,500 mg per day, almost 5 times what most Americans get, due to their eating many of their fish whole, bones and all. For example, their recipe for "Ice Cream" calls for "2 cups moose grease"—not in and of itself high in calcium, but with the addition of "one dressed pike," this Atkins-friendly dessert offers up a respectable 130 mg of calcium per serving. The "unusually rapid bone loss" found in every study ever published on Inuit bone health, however, is blamed on the "acidic effect of a meat diet."

Not only does the near-Atkins level of animal protein in their diet seem to be dissolving their bones, but the near-Atkins level of animal fat leaves the Inuit women's breast milk with some of the highest levels of PCBs in the world. Their blood is swimming with mercury and other toxic heavy metals. "They're at the top of the food chain," says Dr. Russel Shearer, an environmental physical scientist with the Canadian Department of Indian Affairs and Northern Development, and therefore "accumulate the highest levels of these contaminants." In the last edition of his book, Atkins did finally acknowledge the threat posed by the industrial pollutants in animal foods and urged his followers to choose organic, free-range meat.

ATKINS DISTORTED HIS RECORD
ON CHOLESTEROL

Although ketogenic diets have caused a number of "serious, potentially life-threatening complications," perhaps the greatest danger of the Atkins Diet, according to the American Medical Association, lies in the heart.

Atkins claimed that a worsening of cholesterol levels typically occurs only "when carbohydrates are a large part of the diet." We've known this to be false since 1929, when the Institute of American Meatpackers paid to see what would happen if people lived on an all-meat diet. The blood plasma of the unfortunate subjects was so filled with fat it "showed a milkiness," and one of the subjects' cholesterol level shot up to 800!

Slogans like "Reverse heart disease with filet mignon!" notwithstanding, in the head-to-head comparisons of Weight

Watchers, the Zone Diet, the Atkins Diet, and the Ornish Diet (see Chapter 2), Ornish's vegetarian diet was the only one that showed a significant decrease in LDL levels. Even researchers paid by Atkins admit that high-saturated-fat diets like Atkins' tend to increase LDL cholesterol, the single most important risk factor for heart disease, the number one killer in the United States for both men and women.

These researchers have to concede the truth because they publish their work in peer-reviewed scientific journals. Dr. Atkins, though, died without ever publishing a single paper in any scientific journal about anything, and thus had more freedom to bend the truth.

"The truth," Atkins wrote, "is that every one of a score of studies on [very low-carb diets] showed a significant improvement in cholesterol." He accused those who say otherwise of simply not doing their homework. Any claim that cholesterol doesn't significantly improve in "every one of scores of studies" is, he wrote in the last edition, "one of the many examples of untruths being perpetrated because the accusers don't bother to read the scientific literature." He then refers readers to his 1999 recommendation of no less than 17 supplements for the "prevention of cholesterol elevations" on his diet.

But what about his claim that "every one of a score of studies showed a significant improvement in cholesterol"? When the AMA and the American Heart Association question this "fact," is it just because they "don't bother to read the scientific literature"? That statement of his, in the latest edition of his book and in essence repeated to this day on the Atkins website, presents a clear opportunity to test the veracity of his claims. And the truth is almost the exact opposite.

Unfortunately, Dr. Atkins didn't include citations to back up his "score of studies" statement. In fact, when pressed for a list of citations in general, Dr. Atkins told an interviewer that "It and the papers I quoted were in a briefcase I lost some time ago." Researchers have located about a dozen studies, though, that measured the effects of low-carb diets on cholesterol levels. Did they all "show a significant improvement in cholesterol?" No. In fact, with only one exception, every single controlled study showed just the opposite—LDL cholesterol either stagnated or was elevated by a low-carb diet, even in those that showed weight loss.

During active weight loss—any kind of weight loss (whether from chemotherapy, cocaine use, tuberculosis or the Atkins Diet)—cholesterol synthesis temporarily decreases and LDL cholesterol levels *should* go down. However, all the saturated animal fat in the Atkins Diet tends instead to push levels up, and in most studies the bad cholesterol doesn't fall as it should with weight loss. The saturated fat in effect cancelled the benefit one would expect while losing weight and cutting out trans fats. And what happens when people on the Atkins Diet stop losing weight? People can't lose weight forever (Stephen King novels aside). Physicians fear that Atkins dieters' LDL cholesterol levels might then shoot through the roof.

"There is no doubt that you lose weight initially," Dr. Jim Mann, an endocrinology specialist from the University of Otago, New Zealand, told the 2003 meeting of the European Society of Cardiology. "[B]ut there is a grave risk of a dramatic rise in cholesterol levels during the maintenance phase [of the Atkins Diet]. . . . When weight loss is maintained—or, as often happens, there is weight gain [on the Atkins Diet], we have observed that a lot of people experience a rise in cholesterol to levels greater than when they started the diet."

LDL cholesterol levels sometimes became elevated on the Atkins Diet even during the active weight loss stage. One study of women, for example, showed that just two weeks on the Atkins Diet significantly elevated average LDL levels by over 15%. In a trial of men on the Atkins Diet, even though they lost an average of 17 pounds after three months, their LDL cholesterol jumped almost 20%.

The May 2004 *Annals of Internal Medicine* study (see Chapter 4) showed that a third of Atkins dieters suffered a significant increase in LDL cholesterol. The National Cholesterol Education Program recommends aiming for an LDL of less than 100 mg/dl for moderate- to high-risk patients. In the study, one person's LDL shot from an unhealthy 184 to a positively frightening 283 (which means his or her total cholesterol was probably somewhere over 350).

In another clinical trial, despite statistically significant weight loss reported in the Atkins group of the study, every single cardiac risk factor measured had worsened after a year on the Atkins Diet. The investigator concluded: "Those following high-fat [Atkins] diets may have lost weight, but at the price of increased cardiovascular risk factors, including increased LDL cholesterol, increased triglycerides, increased total cholesterol, decreased HDL cholesterol, increased total/HDL cholesterol ratios, and increased homocysteine, Lp(a), and fibrinogen levels. These increased risk factors not only increase the risk of heart disease, but also the risk of strokes, peripheral vascular disease, and blood clots." While the LDL cholesterol levels in the Atkins group increased 6%, in the whole-foods vegetarian group LDL levels were cut in half—dropping 52%. This kind of drop would theoretically make your average American almost heart-attack proof.

When the pro-Atkins journalist who wrote the misleading *New York Times Magazine* piece was asked why he hadn't included the results of this landmark study, which directly contradicted what he wrote in the article, all he could do was accuse the researchers of having made the data up.

It's interesting to note that the one exception—a published study of the Atkins Diet showing a statistically significant reduction in LDL—had no control group, put subjects on cholesterol-lowering supplements, and was funded by the Atkins Corporation itself. Even in that study, though, the drop was modest—only 7% (compared, for example, to the 52% drop on the vegetarian diet)—and didn't include two subjects who quit because their cholesterol levels went out of control.

Yet studies like this have been heralded as a vindication of the Atkins Diet by the mainstream media. As journalist Michael Fumento, co-author of *Fat of the Land*, pointed out, "How peculiar when the most you can say for the best-selling fad-diet book of all time is that it probably doesn't kill people." To which I might add, "in the short term." Based on an analysis of the Atkins Diet, long-term use of the diet is expected to raise coronary heart-disease risk by over 50%. "The late Dr. A," Fumento quips, "still gets an F."

Less often reported in the media is the fact that one of the research subjects placed on the Atkins Diet in the 2003 "vindication" study was hospitalized with chest pain and another died. Similarly, in the widely publicized May 2004 study, less widely publicized was the fact that two people in the low-carb-diet arm of the study couldn't complete the study because they died. One slipped into a coma; the other dropped dead from heart disease. As the director of nutrition at the Harvard School of Medicine has written, "there is still much danger in the widespread fad enthusiasm for these diets."

The Atkins Corporation boasts about the supposed ability of the Atkins Diet to significantly raise the level of HDL, or "good" cholesterol, on a consistent basis. HDL transports cholesterol out of one's arteries to the liver for disposal or recycling. Though in fact only a minority of controlled studies on Atkins-like diets have shown such an effect, it is important to note that the type of HDL increase sometimes seen on these diets is not necessarily healthful. When one eats more garbage (saturated fat and cholesterol) one may need more metabolic garbage trucks (like HDL) to get rid of it. Eating a stick of butter may raise one's HDL, but that doesn't mean chewing one down is good for the heart. In any case, significantly lowering LDL seems more important than significantly raising HDL, though the studies done on low-carb diets typically show neither.

Because of these "well-known hazards of too much saturated fat and cholesterol in most American diets," when Atkins' book was originally published the chair of the nutrition department at Harvard warned physicians that recommending the Atkins Diet "borders on malpractice."

THE PROOF IS IN THE SPECT SCAN

Until the year 2000, all people had to go on in evaluating the impact of the Atkins Diet on the heart were changes in cardiac risk factors like cholesterol. But then a landmark study was published that, for the first (and so far the only) time, actually measured what was happening to people's arteries on this kind of diet. The results were shocking.

Richard Fleming, M.D., an accomplished nuclear cardiologist, enrolled 26 people in a comprehensive study of the effects of diet on cardiac function. Using echocardiograms, he could observe the pumping motion of the heart. And with the latest in nuclear imaging technology—so-called SPECT scans—he was able to actually directly measure the blood flow within the coronary arteries, the blood vessels that bring blood to the heart muscle and allow it to pump. It is when one of these coronary arteries becomes blocked that people have heart attacks.

Fleming put all of the study participants on a whole-foods vegetarian diet, high in carbohydrates and low in saturated fat— the kind that has been proven not only to stop heart disease but, in some cases, to reverse it by opening up clogged arteries. A year later the echocardiograms and SPECT scans were repeated. By that time, however, 10 of his patients admitted that they had, unbeknownst to him, jumped on the low-carb bandwagon and begun following the Atkins Diet or similar diets. All of a sudden, Dr. Fleming had an unparalleled research opportunity dropped in his lap. Here he had extensive imaging of 10 people following a low-carb diet and 16 following a high-carb diet. What would their hearts look like at the end of the year? We can talk about risk factors all we want, but compared to the high-carb group, did the coronary heart disease of the patients following the Atkins Diet improve, worsen, or stay the same?

Those sticking to the whole-foods vegetarian diet showed a reversal of their heart disease as expected. Their partially clogged arteries were literally cleaned out, and blood flow to their hearts through their coronary arteries increased 40%. What happened to those who abandoned the high-carb diet and switched over to the Atkins Diet, chowing down on bunless cheeseburgers and the like? Their condition significantly worsened. All that saturated fat and cholesterol in their diets clogged their arteries further—the blood flow to their hearts was cut 40%. (The blood flow scans have been posted online at http://www.AtkinsExposed.org/atkins/87/Blood_Flow_on_the_Atkins_Diet.htm so people can see the evidence for themselves.) Thus the only study on the Atkins Diet to actually measure arterial blood flow showed that widespread acceptance of diets high in saturated fat could be heralding a future epidemic of fatal heart attacks—validation that, as the Center for Science in the Public Interest wrote, "If you were trying to damage your heart, you couldn't do much better than to eat a cheeseburger." Maybe filet mignon doesn't reverse heart disease after all. According to the American Dietetic Association, the Atkins Diet is "a heart attack waiting to happen."

"We worry about this," explains Dr. James W. Anderson, professor of medicine and clinical nutrition at the University of Kentucky School of Medicine, "because many of the people who love these diets are men aged 40 to 50, who like their meat. They may be five years from their first heart attack. This couldn't be worse for them. Did you know that for 50% of men who die from heart attacks, the fatal attack is their first symptom? They will never know what this diet is doing to them."

Evidence now emerging also suggests that ketogenic diets may "create metabolic derangement conducive to cardiac conduction abnormalities and/or myocardial dysfunction"—in other words, cause other potentially life-threatening heart problems as well. Ketogenic diets may cause a pathological enlargement of the heart called cardiomyopathy, which is reversible, but only if the diet is stopped in time. The Atkins Corporation denies that Dr. Atkins' own cardiomyopathy-induced heart attack, hypertension, and blocked arteries had anything to do with his diet.

SATURATED FAT AND CHOLESTEROL ARE BAD FOR YOU

The Atkins Diet restricts foods that prevent disease and encourages foods that promote disease. No matter what Atkins or other diet books tell people, the balance of evidence clearly shows that intake of saturated animal fat is associated with increased risk of cancer, diabetes, and heart disease. For over 40 years, medical reviews have also shown the detrimental impact of dietary cholesterol consumption. Even independent of the effects on obesity, meat consumption itself has been related to an increased risk of coronary heart disease.

The best dietary strategy to reduce one's risk of dying from the number one killer in the U.S. is to reduce one's consumption of saturated fat and cholesterol. The evidence backing this, according to the American Heart Association, is "overwhelming."

Decreasing America's intake of saturated animal fat is the primary reason why Johns Hopkins, supported by 28 other public health schools, launched the Meatless Mondays campaign, trying to get Americans to cut meat out of their diet at least one day of the week. "The Council," wrote the American Medical Association's Council on Food and Nutrition in their official critique of the Atkins Diet, "is deeply concerned about any diet that advocates an 'unlimited' intake of saturated fats and cholesterol-rich foods."

Dr. Jean Mayer, one of the most noted nutrition figures in history—author of over 750 scientific articles, president of Tufts University, and recipient of 16 honorary degrees—warned people going on "this faddish high-saturated-fat, high-cholesterol [Atkins] diet" that they might be "playing Russian roulette with [their] heart and with [their] blood vessels."

Interestingly, the Atkins Corporation seems like it's already backpedaling. In January 2004, a front-page article in the *New York Times* revealed that the Atkins Corporation was quietly telling people to *restrict* their bacon and butter intake, urging them to keep saturated fat intake under 20% of calories. Though nearly every major health organization in the world recommends less than half that amount, Atkins' change in policy does at least show that the Atkins Corporation may be recognizing some of the dangers of its diet.

The Atkins Corporation claimed in the article that their saturated fat guideline was nothing new and that Atkins never said people could eat as much meat as they wanted. They blamed the media for just misconstruing the Atkins Diet as an eat-as-much-meat-as-you-want diet. Really? *Dr. Atkins' Diet Revolution* states, "There is no limit to the amount of [any kind of meat in any quantity] you can eat. . . ." You eat as *much* as you want, as *often* as you want" (emphasis in original). In fact Atkins specifically boasts in the 1999 edition that his diet "sets no limit on the amount of food you can eat." Maybe the media got it right.

The director of research and education at Atkins Nutritionals claims that "Saturated fat isn't as much of an issue when carbohydrates are controlled; it's only dangerous in excess when carbs are high." Dr. Frank M. Sacks, a professor of cardiovascular disease prevention at the Harvard School of Public Health, scoffed at such a claim. "What they are saying is ridiculous," he said. The revision down to 20% saturated fat, he added, "has nothing to do with science; it has to do with public relations and politics."

CLOSING OFF HIS HEART TO THE ATKINS DIET

One can still go to the Atkins website, though, and read how innocuous saturated fat is. One reader asks, "Is it OK for me to consume more than 20% of my calories in the form of saturated fat?" The answer given is "Absolutely."

With this kind of advice, 53-year-old businessman Jody Gorran stayed on the Atkins Diet and continued to recommend it to his friends, even though his cholesterol had shot up 50%. Before starting the Atkins Diet, his cholesterol was excellent, he had no history of heart disease, and an unrelated CT scan showed that his coronary arteries were clean.

For Jody Gorran, it took two years on the Atkins Diet before the crushing chest pain started. By then, one of his coronary arteries was 99% blocked and his heart function was suffering for it. He underwent an immediate cardiac catheterization and stent placement that may have saved his life. Otherwise, according to his cardiologist, Gorran might well have had a massive heart attack and died within a short period of time. Mr. Gorran is now suing the Atkins Corporation, alleging that it "knew, or should have known" that what it was saying about its diet and heart disease risk were false. He is trying to get the corporation to include warning labels on its books, website, and products that a low-carbohydrate diet "may be hazardous to your health—check with your physician."

This is not the first time Atkins has been sued. When *Dr. Atkins' Diet Revolution* first came out, a million-dollar class action suit was brought against Atkins and his publisher to recover medical expenses incurred by the diet's side effects. A Brooklyn assemblyman on the Atkins Diet who nearly died of a heart attack sued Atkins and the publisher for producing a book "without regard to the safety, truth or accuracy of the statements contained in the book." The book *Nutrition Cultism* cites three suits against Atkins; the cases were each settled out of court in favor of the plaintiffs.

"The point is," Gorran said in an NBC News interview, "Dr. Atkins lied to the public. He didn't care. For his ego or for corporate greed, that's what this thing's about." On *Good Morning America*, Gorran pointed out that "A successful diet has to be more than simply losing weight. . . . A successful diet should not kill you."

RACHEL

Most people aren't able to remain on the Atkins Diet long enough to develop osteoporosis, kidney damage or hardening of the arteries. Sixteen-year-old Rachel Elizabeth Huskey only lasted seven weeks.

Rachel had a crush on a boy in her church. So she started the Atkins Diet to lose weight. In part because she was so nauseated on the diet, she lost 16 pounds. She hoped that being thinner would make her more popular at school. After a brief carbohydrate relapse, she began again "very strictly." Eight days into this effort, Rachel collapsed without warning in her history class. And then she died. Frenzied attempts to resuscitate her failed. Her doctors blame the Atkins Diet.

The kidney uses minerals such as potassium and calcium to help rid the body of toxins like ketones. People on the Atkins Diet are urinating these minerals away. And critically low blood levels of these electrolytes can lead to fatal cardiac arrhythmias— lethal heart rhythms. Rachel was on the Atkins Diet at the time·

of her death from cardiac arrhythmia and was found on autopsy to have critically low blood levels of both potassium and calcium. Rachel was previously in good health and had no history of any medical problems.

After ruling out other potential causes, the medical team of child health specialists that investigated her death couldn't help but conclude in their published report, "Sudden cardiac death of an adolescent during dieting," that the Atkins Diet was the most likely cause of her death.

The chief executive of the Atkins Corporation denied there was a link between the diet and Rachel's death, but implied she should have consulted her doctor before starting the diet. In fact, concern over just such an event led the director of the nutrition department at the esteemed Cleveland Clinic to declare that for people on the Atkins Diet, "Careful monitoring of electrolytes is absolutely essential. . . ." Those who aren't professionally monitored on this kind of diet "are at the greatest risk for dangerous complications."

Dr. Paul Robinson, the director of adolescent medicine at the University of Missouri, who was involved in the investigation of Rachel's death, is afraid that "we're having lots of near misses that we don't know about. . . . You wonder whether there are other people dying and we don't know about it."

"Is the diet safe for teenagers?" Dr. Atkins was asked in an interview. He replied, "The [Atkins] diet is safe for every overweight human being from the age of 18 months. . . ." Guided by this doctrine, the Atkins Corporation is trying to make inroads into schools. "I frankly think it's scandalous," said the director of the Yale Prevention Research Center, "really very dangerous."

One would think that a teenager collapsing and dying after just days on the diet might have ruined the public's appetite for Atkins, but Rachel's death was scarcely reported in the American press. When her parents held a press conference to tell their story for the first time and warn others that Atkins "killed our little girl," it was reported in London, Scotland, New Zealand, Australia, and South Africa. But out of the 34 reports that made it into the papers around the world about the Missouri teen, only three appeared in the United States. Despite repeated warnings from the American Heart Association, enthusiasm for the Atkins Diet did not seem to wane.

While tending her daughter's immaculately kept grave, Rachel's mom told a reporter her thoughts on the diet: "I want people to know you can actually die doing something as stupid as this."

DOWN ON ATKINS DOWN UNDER

Like the tobacco industry, as bad press mounts here in the United States, the Atkins Corporation is exporting its product overseas. In August 2004, for example, it hired a public relations firm to, as one newspaper headline put it, "invade Latin America."

Australia appears to be one of the few nations in which action is actually being taken at a state level. The Victorian Health Minister, supported by the Australian Heart Foundation and the Australian Medical Association, issued a warning to alert people to the dangers of the Atkins Diet and other high-fat fad diets. The government is warning the public about the potential short-term effects—constipation, dehydration, bad breath, low energy and poor concentration—and potential long-term effects, such as the increased likelihood of cancer, heart disease, depression, and osteoporosis. "When we know something is bad for people, like smoking," the health minister explained, "then we let people know what the health risks are."

Initially, the government will distribute educational materials in doctors' waiting rooms, gyms, and universities, probably followed by advertising in bus shelters and in the media. Australia's chief physician urged all governments to follow suit.

The Atkins empire said that this was the first government to launch a public health campaign against them. Health Canada did propose to ban "low-carb" product claims, and the British government did issue a warning against low-carbohydrate diets, saying they were "bad for your health," though it didn't specifically name Atkins. The "U.S. Federal Government officials," Atkins corporate representatives said, "had a much more positive response. . . ." Perhaps "low-carb" foods aren't a $30 billion business down under.

ONLY UNDER MONTHLY CLINICAL SUPERVISION

In a 1979 medical journal article entitled "Bizarre and unusual diets," the authors warned that the Atkins Diet's safety was so questionable that it should "only be followed under medical supervision." But what do doctors know about nutrition? Even though the United States Congress mandated that nutrition become an integrated component of medical education, as of 2004, less than half of all U.S. medical schools have a single mandatory course in nutrition. That explains the results of a study published in the *American Journal of Clinical Nutrition* that pitted doctors against patients head-to-head in a test of basic nutrition knowledge. The patients won. People off the street seem to know more about nutrition than their doctors.

In any case, despite their relative ignorance of nutrition, doctors can still do their job and monitor for adverse health effects. Since "[t]he Atkins program falls short in . . . warning dieters," another review of popular weight loss diets points out, patients must therefore "be monitored by a physician" to ensure their safety. According to the chair of the nutrition department at Harvard Medical School, people on the Atkins Diet "should be monitored for orthostatic hypotension . . . dizziness, headaches, fatigue, irritability, gout, and kidney failure." And laboratory work should include "blood tests (glucose, blood urea nitrogen, sodium, potassium, chloride, and bicarbonate), urinalysis (specific gravity, pH, protein, and acetone), and a lipid profile. Vital signs . . . should be monitored at least monthly during a low-carbohydrate weight-loss program."

The Atkins Diet is already estimated to cost $10,000–$20,000 per year for food and supplements. Perhaps one should add the expense of monthly doctor visits as well, or risk the consequences.

CHAPTER 6

THE SAFER ALTERNATIVE

······················

WHERE ATKINS DESERVED CREDIT

ONCE, WHEN DR. DEAN ORNISH WAS BEING INTERVIEWED ON *Dateline NBC,* his interviewer swore that he had lost 50 pounds on the Atkins Diet, ate a steak every day, and felt great. He asked Ornish, "How bad could it be?" When Ornish turned the tables and questioned the host, it came out that before going on Atkins he'd been living off French fries, fried onion rings, cheesecake, and at least five soft drinks per day, every day. He had since cut all those out and started exercising religiously. Ornish pointed out that he was probably feeling better in spite of the steak, not because of it.

While Atkins used to tell people to eat unlimited quantities of hydrogenated shortening like Crisco, thankfully he reversed his position and now warns about the "dangers of trans fats." Just cutting out deep-fried foods (most often fried in 100% vegetable—and 100% *hydrogenated*—oil) from one's diet should alone improve one's cholesterol profile. Atkins also encouraged everyone to cut out caffeine and eat more heart-healthy nuts and omega-3 fatty acids, and did consider daily exercise a critical, "non-negotiable" component of his plan.

Anyone completely cutting out sugary soda, pastries, ice cream, cookies, cake, candy, kids' cereals, and Snackwells is probably going to feel better. But do we need a 300-page diet book to tell us that? Anything that can give Krispy Kreme's corporate profits that glazed look is a good thing for America's health.

For those who don't remember, Snackwells were Nabisco's line of low-fat and fat-free junk food that rocketed from zero to a billion dollars in revenues in four short years, in effect becoming America's most popular cookie. When Snackwells' fat-free Devil's Food Cookie Cakes first appeared, demand was so high that Nabisco had to ration them out to stores and fights broke out between shoppers, forcing store managers to keep boxes of the cookies under lock and key.

People were mistaking low-fat for low-calorie. The intention of the government's recommendation to cut down on fat was to get people to cut down on items like meat and switch to foods that are *naturally* low in fat—like beans, whole grains, fruits and vegetables. These don't have much of a profit margin, however, so the food industry took advantage of the new guidelines to market low-fat junk food like Snackwells cookies, swapping fat for sugar. Each cookie was basically just white flour and two spoonfuls of sugar. Even bags of jelly beans started boasting "fat-free." A similar phenomenon is now happening with low-carb junk food. A new Atkins-friendly ice cream, for example, has almost twice the calories of regular ice cream (and of course twice the fat). "It's Snackwells all over again," noted one *WebMD Medical News* article. Junk food—low-fat or low-carb—is still junk food.

People also may feel better on the Atkins Diet because Atkins tells people to stop drinking cow's milk. Even the National Dairy Council admits that literally most people on the planet are lactose-intolerant (and may not even know it). That change alone should make a segment of the people trying the Atkins

Diet feel better. In addition to those who are lactose-intolerant, other easy born-again Atkins converts might be those with an actual dairy allergy or the one out of every few hundred Americans who is allergic to wheat.

Even at his strictest, Atkins "allowed" two small salads a day. Although they can only be a cup of "loosely" packed greens each, that's sadly more salad than many non-Atkins-dieting Americans may get, so Atkins dieters following this recommendation may feel some benefit from that. Atkins even recommended eating one's greens organic, dark, and leafy. Then again, the "spinach salad" recipe in his 1972 book calls for an entire pound of bacon and 5 eggs. No croutons, of course—"use crumbled fried pork rinds instead."

THE ANSWERS ARE *NO* AND *NO*

There seem to be two Atkins Diets: the one that's described in Atkins' books (particularly in later editions) and the one the public *thinks* is described in his books. How many Atkins dieters, for example, only eat free-range, organic bacon?

A recent study of 11,000 people found that only one in four of those claiming to be on a low-carb diet were actually significantly cutting carbs at all. Another survey, commissioned by former Surgeon General C. Everett Koop's organization Shape Up America!, found that most people claiming to be on Atkins, or another of the low-carb fad diets, didn't even seem to know where carbs were found. Most didn't know, for example, that tomatoes are high in carbs. Thankfully, about half of them didn't know apples had a lot of carbs, and one in six even thought steak was a carbohydrate. This may be one of the reasons why we haven't seen even higher rates of serious side effects—there may be a relatively small number of people actually following the diet. Thankfully, most people on Atkins are actually *not* on Atkins.

Despite the softening of his stance on whole grains and many vegetables in the latest edition of his book, Atkins still made saturated-fat-laden meat and cheese the centerpiece of his diet. The Atkins Diet therefore remains dangerous even when "used as directed."

Isn't it possible to do the Atkins Diet healthfully? Isn't there some way to modify it to make it safer? Those exact questions were asked of the editors at the *Tufts University Health and Nutrition Letter* by one of the university's vice presidents. After trying their best, the editorial staff at the *Tufts Letter* couldn't help but conclude, "So, as to whether it's possible to follow the Atkins Diet healthfully or tweak it to make it safe and healthful, the answers are *no* and *no*" (emphasis in original).

TOO GOOD TO BE TRUE

What kind of diet can cause birth defects? Or blindness? Or require 65 supplements? Or monthly medical checkups, where the monitoring of electrolytes is considered "absolutely essential"? Is it too much to ask that one's diet facilitate instead of debilitate physical activity? (Here in Boston there has yet to be a night of pork-rind loading before the Marathon.) What kind of diet may require prescriptions to deal with the side effects? What kind of diet has side effects at all?

Rational people go on irrational diets because "they're desperate," says Kelly Brownell, director of Yale University's Center for Eating and Weight Disorders. "If you're a person with an overweight body living in a thin-obsessed world . . . something that offers a miracle is highly attractive."

The director of nutrition at the Center for Science in the Public Interest is dumbfounded that the high-fat regimes have caught on. "With all the evidence that saturated fat promotes heart disease, it's almost unbelievable to me that people could successfully tell people to eat bacon, eggs, ground beef, cheese, and cream," she says. "It really shows that people care more about how they look than how healthy they are."

Obesity shouldn't be a cosmetic or moral issue, but it does remain a health issue. Obesity, as defined by the Institute of Medicine, is "an important chronic degenerative disease that debilitates individuals and kills prematurely." Obesity continues to contribute to hundreds of thousands of deaths in the U.S. every year. Losing weight is important, but the goal should be to lose weight in a way that enhances health rather than harms it. People also use cocaine, amphetamines, and tobacco to control their weight—not health-promoting solutions to the problem.

Consumer Guide concluded in 1974 that the Atkins Diet "owes its appeal, like pornography, to the naughtiness of the approach, to the titillation we all feel in doing something which we think is not right." Diet gurus like Atkins—the "bad boy of diets"—gave people what they wanted to hear, says James Hill, director of the University of Colorado Center for Human Nutrition. Asks one Atkins disciple, "Who wouldn't like a diet that allows fried eggs and bacon and all the steak you can eat?" "But what people want to hear," Dr. Hill adds, "is killing them."

ATKINS IS BASED ON A HALF-TRUTH

Despite U.S. attempts to stall and sabotage the World Health Organization's report on diet (using similar tactics as when they opposed the WHO's Framework Convention on Tobacco Control), in May 2004 the WHO Global Strategy on Diet, Physical Activity, and Health was unanimously endorsed by all 192 Member States of the United Nations. The report blames the growing pandemic of global chronic disease in part on "greater saturated fat intake (mostly from animal sources), reduced intakes of complex carbohydrates and dietary fiber, and reduced fruit and vegetable intakes." In other words, they blame the global epidemic of obesity, cancer, heart disease, and diabetes on exactly the kind of diet Atkins' books recommend. As the *Harvard Health Letter* put it, the Atkins Diet simply "is not a healthy way to eat." The World Health Organization is calling for limiting the consumption of saturated animal fats and "increasing the consumption of fruits, vegetables, legumes [beans, peas and lentils], whole grains, and nuts."

The evidence to support their position is "overwhelming." After 11 years following 11,000 people, for example, researchers found that eating whole grains may help people live longer. That did not seem to be the case for refined grains, though. And the Atkins Diet is based on that half-truth.

Atkins was right in going "against the grain" in the case of refined carbohydrates like white flour and sugar. But he was wrong to restrict good carbs—the carbs found in whole, unrefined foods, like those recommended in the WHO's report: "fruits, vegetables, legumes, whole grains, and nuts." A bunless burger is not the answer to a fat-free doughnut.

While jelly beans and Wonder Bread are not health-promoting foods, that doesn't mean one has to switch to pork rinds and bacon. Let's not throw the wheat germ out with the wheat.

YOU CAN HAVE YOUR CARBS AND EAT THEM TOO

What evidence do we have that "good" carbs are good? Every single long-term prospective study ever performed on the foods that the Atkins Diet restricts—fruits, vegetables, nuts and whole grains—shows that these foods protect people from the nation's biggest killer: heart disease. Harvard studied 75,000 women for a decade, and the results suggest that the more whole grains people eat—like brown rice and whole wheat bread—the lower their risk of having a heart attack. Harvard studied 40,000 men for a decade and suggested that eating whole grains may cut one's risk of developing diabetes by more than half. The only thing wrong with whole grains, perhaps, is that they may not sell as many books.

Atkins seemed to think that fruit was the worst thing since sliced bread. Fruit consumption alone, however, has been linked to lower rates of numerous cancers and may reduce heart disease mortality, cancer, and total mortality. The World Health Organization blames low fruit and vegetable consumption for literally millions of deaths worldwide. Everyone should eat more fruits and vegetables—as if their lives depended on it.

The National Cancer Institute's recommendation is now up to *nine* servings of fruits and vegetables every day. While Atkins preached to restrict fruit and vegetable intake, what Americans really need is more fruits and veggies, not less.

LOSE WEIGHT WITHOUT LOSING YOUR HEALTH—OR YOUR LIFE

Lifelong weight control is a marathon; fad diets are sold on the 100-yard dash. The U.C. Berkeley School of Public Health's number one rated newsletter gives the "Bottom Line" on Atkins: "Bottom Line: If you follow the Atkins Diet, you will lose weight—but it could be dangerous beyond a few weeks. All fad diets get you to cut down on calories, usually by limiting the kinds of food you can eat, so of course you lose weight. Most, like the Atkins Diet, deny that 'calories count,' but nonetheless trick you into cutting way down on calories by distracting you with strange rules and psychological/biochemical babble. As with all crash diets, keeping the weight off is the hard part. Virtually all crash dieters eventually gain the weight back, unless they learn the basics of healthy eating, which crash diets do not teach." Diets are not something to be followed for days or weeks or months. They should form the basis of everyday food choices for the rest of one's life.

So what are the "basics of healthy eating?" According to the

American Dietetics Association, "The overwhelming majority of studies reported to date, including both epidemiological and laboratory approaches, suggest that eating carbohydrate-rich foods such as vegetables, fruits, legumes and whole grains, and limiting saturated fat intake, over a lifetime, is associated with substantially reduced risk for vascular disease and some cancers." It may be no coincidence that the longest-living people in the world, even by some accounts outlasting the Okinawan Japanese, are the California Seventh-day Adventist vegetarians.

Every study of the Atkins Diet over six months in duration found that the Atkins Diet failed to significantly outperform the exact diet Atkins blamed for America's obesity epidemic. Why not, then, choose a healthier diet?

Fewer than 20% of Americans trying to lose weight follow what's considered the optimal diet plan for weight control, the one proven to be safe and effective for losing weight, keeping the weight off, and promoting health—a diet low in saturated animal fats and high in fruits, vegetables and high-fiber carbohydrates like beans and whole grains. How convenient that the most healthful diet also seems to be the one most successful in controlling one's weight.

To lose weight, one can cut down on calorie intake by restricting the amount of food one eats, or one can transition away from eating junk food—foodstuffs long on calories but short on nutrition—and toward eating food that is nutrient-dense but relatively calorie-dilute: foods like fruits, vegetables, beans and whole grains. One can add nuts to the list as well, since, despite their caloric density, a 2003 review concluded that eating nuts every day might actually help one maintain or even lose weight. People placed on nutrient-dense, calorie-dilute plant-based diets tend not to complain of hunger but of having "too much food."

The healthy alternative to the Atkins Diet is not a fat-free diet, but a *fad*-free diet. "Nobody wants to hear this," groaned Dr.

James W. Anderson in an interview. Anderson is a professor of medicine and clinical nutrition at the University of Kentucky School of Medicine. "People lose weight [on the Atkins Diet], at least in the short term. I am not arguing with that. But this is absolutely the worst diet you could imagine for long-term obesity, heart disease, and some forms of cancer. If you wanted to find one diet to ruin your health, you couldn't find one worse than Atkins."

The optimal diet is one centered around good carbohydrates (unrefined), good fats (like nuts), and the best sources of protein, which, according to the Harvard School of Medicine, are "beans, nuts, grains, and other vegetable sources of protein." In other words, we don't have to mortgage our health in order to lose weight. By eating a whole-food, plant-based diet people can control their weight without risking their health—or their lives.

FADING FAD

The momentum to educate the American public is growing. The week after my website was launched, the Partnership for Essential Nutrition, a new broad-based coalition of nearly a dozen nonprofit consumer, nutrition and public health organizations, escalated its efforts to combat the growing misinformation about carbohydrates.

Thankfully, the fad seems to be fading once again. Based on surveys of thousands of American adults, the low-carb craze seems to have peaked around January 2004 and is expected to continue to peter out, according to food-industry analysts at Morgan Stanley. Most industry analysts and consultants are now suggesting that this latest low-carb wave is indeed a passing fad. According to *Fortune* magazine, data show that the number of Americans on a low-carb diet has dropped 25% since January.

The American public finally seems to be waking up to the

truth. In one survey, for example, fewer than one in five consumers surveyed said they would even consider purchasing a low-carb product. Reasons given for not going low-carb included the belief that low-carb diets were neither healthy nor effective.

We seem to have come full circle, from celebrities boasting about Atkins to celebrities now threatening to sue anyone who repeats allegations that they were ever following the Atkins Diet in the first place. Even cattlemen are starting to get worried as demand for beef starts to slip. A backlash seems to be brewing in the business world with a slew of advertisements poking fun at the low-carb fad.

Declining demand is also starting to affect the low-carb corporate bottom line. Food giants clamored onto the bandwagon, *Maclean's* noted, "just as its wheels started to fall off." Food manufacturers are being stuck with backlogs of low-carb products, and a number of planned low-carb lines have been scuttled due to disappointing sales. Business journals publish articles with titles like this one from *Forbes Magazine*: "A low-carb retailing disaster: A pack of entrepreneurs chased the low-carb dream— over a cliff" with increasing frequency. "There's been a bloodbath in the industry," admits the head of Lowcarbiz, a low-carb business association. The *Wall Street Journal* calls this phenomenon the "food-fad effect."

A year ago, the Atkins empire couldn't crank out products fast enough; now, retailers are discounting them. By the second quarter of 2004, low-carb product sales growth was cut in half. Layoffs at the Atkins Corporation started in September 2004.

Food industry researchers conclude that consumers seem to be finally wising up to the health risks. "It defied logic," said one industry expert, "Bacon is better for you than orange juice. Yeah, right." Or as one Wall Street analyst explained, "Have you ever tried low-carb bread?"

THE ATKINS CORPORATION RESPONDS

·····················

Re: Your Statements Concerning Atkins and Use of Atkins Trademarks

Dear Dr. Greger:
This is on behalf of Atkins Nutritionals, Inc. ("Atkins") in regard to certain statements appearing on your website located at www.AtkinsFacts.org. . . .

ON AUGUST 3, 2004, THE LEGAL DEPARTMENT OF THE ATKINS Corporation sent me a letter threatening to sue me for speaking out against the Atkins Diet on my website www.AtkinsFacts.org. They claim my website "impinges on Atkins' rights" by making "defamatory" statements that "continue to harm Atkins' reputation and cause injury to Atkins."

This is typical corporate behavior. The tobacco industry, for example, accused public health advocates of "defaming" Philip Morris. Though millions of children have been poisoned by lead paint in the United States, the Lead Industries Association once threatened to sue a public health advocate for daring to say that "lead paint was bad to eat."

I am not the only one Atkins has tried to silence (see the Introduction). Just as Dr. Atkins once sued Nathan Pritikin, the Atkins Corporation is now threatening me for AtkinsFacts.org (now AtkinsExposed.org to avoid any confusion with the Atkins corporate website).

I refused to be bullied into silence, however, and posted the company's entire legal threat letter online for all to see, accompanied by a point-by-point rebuttal. Thankfully, under law the truth is considered an absolute defense against defamation.

Below are the major points addressed in the corporation's letter (quoted in indented italics) and my rebuttal. To read their letter in full, as well as my complete rebuttal, visit www.AtkinsExposed.org.

- **AtkinsFacts.org Relies on "Mere Opinions"**

  In the face of [the overwhelming] medical evidence, most claims on your website constitute either exaggerated or scientifically undemonstrated statements, mere opinions from medical professionals or organizations. . . .

"Mere opinions" from medical professionals or organizations? This is exactly the tack the tobacco industry took. When the American Cancer Society and others condemned smoking, the tobacco corporations said that the smoking/lung cancer link was "mere opinion," "exaggerated," and "undemonstrated" as well. Now that the American Cancer Society has similarly warned against low-carb diets, your response seems the same.

The official published statements of medical organizations are not "mere opinion." The American Medical Association uses 56 citations to back up its condemnation of the Atkins Diet. The

American Heart Association uses 54 in its warning about low-carb diets. The chair of Harvard's nutrition department uses 35. The U.S. Department of Agriculture uses 198. The American Dietetic Association used 16 in its warning about the Atkins Diet. To dismiss the reasoned, independent, objective evaluations of these organizations as "mere opinions" is to devalue the scientific process.

I think it is reasonable to hold the "mere opinions" of the American Cancer Society, the American Institute for Cancer Research, the American Kidney Fund, the American Obesity Association, the American Association of Diabetes Educators, the Center for Science in the Public Interest, the Cleveland Clinic, the Mayo Clinic, Cornell University, Johns Hopkins University, Northwestern University, Tufts University, the University of California at Davis, the Yale-Griffin Prevention Research Center, and Jean Mayer (probably the most widely acclaimed nutritionist in American history) as more compelling than the "mere opinions" of Atkins Nutritionals, Inc.

- **AtkinsFacts.org Ignores "the Overwhelming Weight of the Evidence"**

  As you are undoubtedly aware, your position that the ANA [Atkins Nutritional Approach, i.e. the Atkins Diet] presents serious health risks is at odds with the overwhelming weight of the evidence.

  There is, in fact, an overwhelming weight of evidence, but it points to the opposite of what you're claiming. AtkinsFacts.org is hardly alone in condemning the Atkins Diet out of fear for the public's health. The American Cancer Society, the American Heart Association, the American Dietetic Association, and the American Medical Association all have publicly come out against

Atkins-like diets and warned of serious potential health risks. Literally dozens of medical and nutritional authorities have attempted to educate the public about the very real dangers associated with diets like yours. Their position statements are reprinted in full in my "Expert Opinions" section at http://www.AtkinsExposed.org/atkins/22/Opinions.htm.

- **AtkinsFacts.org Ignores the 34 Studies "Supporting Atkins"**

  In fact, as documented on the Atkins website, . . . there are currently no fewer than thirty-four studies demonstrating the weight loss and other health benefits—and absence of adverse health effects—of a low-carbohydrate diet.

In citing studies you claim support your diet, you cast your position as scientific, though no major governmental or non-profit medical, nutrition, or science-based organization in the world agrees with this characterization. A 2004 review in the *Journal of the American College of Cardiology* concluded that the Atkins Diet "runs counter to all the current evidence-based dietary recommendations."

Apparently, out of literally hundreds of published reports on low-carbohydrate diets, the Atkins Corporation can only find 34 that support its position. For that matter, there are 34 studies demonstrating the health benefits of cigarette smoking. There are also 34 studies showing benefits from thalidomide. If you go to the website of the Asbestos Institute you can find 34 studies downplaying the risks of asbestos. Or you can go to a chemical manufacturer's website and find 34 studies that downplay the risk of arsenic-treated wood for children's playgrounds (a practice now banned by the EPA). On a website supported by pesticide makers you can find no fewer than 34 studies downplaying the risks of DDT.

While the Philip Morris Corporation can wave around more than a hundred studies showing health benefits from smoking, this doesn't mean that smoking is good for you. What it means is that one can cherry-pick data to argue almost any position. This is a classic tobacco corporation tactic. Like tobacco, asbestos, and chemical companies, you seem to be willing to distort the scientific record by cherry-picking statistics to produce the illusion that the balance of evidence is on your side.

So, even if there were 34 studies published in peer-reviewed scientific journals supporting the Atkins Diet, independent systematic reviews of the entirety of scientific evidence support neither smoking nor the Atkins Diet for one's health. Still, since these studies seem to be the basis of your defense, let me examine them in greater detail.

Over a Quarter of the "Research Studies" Are Not Even Published

First of all, 9 of the 34 cited studies "supporting Atkins" are not published studies at all, but merely abstracts (brief paragraphs written about unpublished studies) presented at meetings, which in general, wrote an editor of the *New England Journal of Medicine*, "must be presumed to be unreliable sources of public information." This is another tried and true tobacco industry strategy.

Information provided in abstracts is considered "of little use to the general medical community" because the information presented is "limited and insufficient to allow critical appraisal of the work." "Abstracts of papers presented at meetings," concluded a review in the *Journal of the American Medical Association*, "have been seen as an untrustworthy basis for scientific communication."

Less than half of studies presented as abstracts may ever be published at all. As the *New England Journal of Medicine* editorialized, "Presumably, most of the other papers were so flawed or so unimportant that either they were never submitted for publication or they were rejected as a result of peer review." If and when the studies are published, one finds that the abstracts may routinely overstate the case.

The purpose of meeting abstracts is to stimulate dialogue, not to support a position or product. A past editor of the *New England Journal of Medicine* considered abstracts so unreliable that he felt that news media shouldn't even report research findings presented only in abstract form. As one medical journal editor concluded, the guiding principle when considering abstract credibility is *caveat emptor*.

The "Uniform Requirements for Manuscripts Submitted to Biomedical Journals" drafted by the International Committee of Medical Journal Editors and in use by over 500 journals specifically admonishes researchers to "Avoid using abstracts as references." The validity of abstracts is so questionable that some medical journals entirely prohibit authors from even citing them. Yet abstracts make up over a quarter of the "research studies" that you use as references to "support" the Atkins Diet.

Others Were Published in a Journal Founded by an Atkins Spokesman

The remaining studies were published in peer-reviewed journals. Four of these "peer-reviewed" studies, however, were published in a journal I had never heard of called *Metabolic Syndrome and Related Disorders*. When I couldn't find it in Harvard's medical library, which boasts 26,000 serial titles, or indeed anywhere in the medical mecca of Boston, I became curious.

I called the publisher. I asked them if in fact a single medical library in the country carried their journal. They confirmed that Atkins Nutritionals, Inc. had an active subscription, but the only medical library that seemed to carry their journal, they said, was one in Alabama. I checked. They don't. In fact, the journal isn't even indexed by the U.S. National Library of Medicine's Index Medicus or any of the other major medical databases, which contain over 12,000 titles. I clearly had more detective work to do.

It turns out the journal was founded by Dr. Eric Freedland, a member and self-described representative of THINCS, The International Network of Cholesterol Skeptics. The Cholesterol Skeptics deny that cholesterol and saturated fat cause heart disease.

Dr. Freedland, founder and still associate editor of *Metabolic Syndrome and Related Disorders*, has not only been a featured speaker at conferences sponsored by the Atkins Foundation but reportedly was the president of your Atkins at Home program, where followers pay $1,000 a month to get Atkins meals delivered to their door. Dr. Freedland has also been reportedly listed as one of your official spokesmen.

Is it a coincidence that the journal "dedicated its premiere issue to the life's work of Dr. Atkins"? The Atkins issue was organized by Dr. Freedland, who wrote the issue's "Tribute to Robert C. Atkins, M.D." and dedicated it to Atkins' memory. "I have had the privilege of personally knowing Dr. Atkins," Freedman wrote, "and it is indeed sad to lose a loved one. . . ." He wrote about the responsibility to "carry the torch and continue his vision."

This is the "prestigious," "authoritative, peer-reviewed journal" that you boast published research supporting Atkins?—a journal reportedly founded by one of your paid spokesmen? The journal even featured a commentary by Atkins' widow. Veronica Atkins admitted that her late husband had never published anything in any peer-reviewed medical journal but said she was "delighted to be able to say that I have now accomplished this on his behalf!"

Most of the Studies Were Published by Atkins-Funded Researchers

Speaking of those paid by Atkins, most of the 34 cited articles were published by Atkins-funded researchers—those given money by you directly or through the Dr. Robert C. Atkins Foundation. Another six of the studies did not reveal the source of their funding (less than half of major scientific and medical journals require disclosure of conflicts of interest).

As you know, the Atkins Foundation was started by Dr. Atkins and has given millions of dollars to researchers to, in the words of co-founder Veronica Atkins, "prove Dr. Atkins right."

Corporations have had a long history of misrepresenting science. Asbestos corporations fund, publish, and cite studies that downplay the risks of asbestos. Chemical companies fund, publish, and cite studies that downplay the risks of their products. Tobacco corporations fund, publish, and cite studies that downplay the risks of tobacco. It is not surprising that you, the billion-dollar Atkins Corporation, fund, publish, and cite studies that downplay the risks of your product, the Atkins Diet.

Corporate sponsorship can overtly or covertly influence the conduct and publication of research in a variety of ways. In particular, investigators may fear that future funding may be denied if they publish data unfavorable to the hand that feeds them. A study showed that the odds that researchers with tobacco industry affiliations would conclude that secondhand smoke was harmless, for example, are almost a hundred times higher than the odds that non-affiliated researchers would come to such a conclusion.

To combat the wealth of evidence showing that cigarette smoking caused lung cancer, U.S. tobacco companies formed the Council for Tobacco Research ostensibly to "fund independent scientific research on the health effects of smoking." Not surprisingly, though, internal documents showed that their true aim was to create studies specifically designed to produce data to support their arguments. The Atkins Corporation seems to be taking tips from the tobacco industry.

You claim that you are relying on "sound science." This is the same name Philip Morris's public relations firm gave to a campaign to downplay the risks of cigarette smoke and "manipulate the scientific standards of proof for the corporate interests of their clients." Your attempt to recruit doctors into your "Atkins Physicians Council" to downplay the risks of the Atkins Diet is reminiscent of Philip Morris's secret campaign, code-named "Project Whitecoat."

Though the products of both industries have been condemned by the American Cancer Society, the American Heart Association, and the American Medical Association, you and the tobacco corporations both built up networks of scientists sympathetic to your position, funded independent organizations to give an impression of legitimate, unbiased science, and organized symposiums to publish non-peer-reviewed research and give your funded research, in the words of one tobacco executive, "a deep fragrance of academia."

Evidence shows that tobacco corporation-affiliated researchers routinely ignored data that didn't support their position. Might not Atkins-affiliated researchers be guilty of the same thing?

Atkins Responds to Criticism "Who Pays the Piper Calls the Tune"

You deny that your funding influences the results. "Speaking of funding," Dr. Atkins himself wrote, "the media jumped on the fact that the Dr. Robert C. Atkins Foundation funded the study, implying that the results were therefore suspect. Get real! Who do they think is funding the vast majority of funding for drug research? Pharmaceutical companies, of course. Does that mean that all research on prescription drugs is equally suspect?"

In choosing the pharmaceutical industry, Dr. Atkins seems to have picked the wrong business to exemplify lack of funding-source influence. According to World Health Organization director Jonathan Quick, "researchers who publish or communicate results unfriendly to the [drug company] sponsors have faced intimidation, attempts to discredit them professionally, and legal threats to recover 'lost sales.' "

Citing drug manufacturers' profit motive for skewing reports of their drugs' safety, an editorial in the *Lancet* reads, "Tobacco is not the only aspect of medicine open to twisted corporate communications strategies. . . . All policymakers must be vigilant to the possibility of research data being manipulated by corporate bodies and of scientific colleagues being seduced by the material charms of industry. Trust is no defense against an aggressively deceptive corporate sector."

Highly statistically significant associations have consistently been found between sources of funding and outcome of drug studies. One medical professor looked at over a hundred studies of new drugs sponsored by the manufacturer. Not a *single* one found their drug inferior to the competitor's. Other studies have found the same uncanny "coincidence."

Corporations manipulate funded research in a variety of ways. Companies may be selective in publishing results, for example, and "may delay or not publish unfavorable results at all." If the researchers find negative results or adverse effects, the corporation can just suppress the truth. "Withholding the publication of unfavorable results," according to the *Journal of the American Medical Association*, "is not uncommon."

The bottom line is that whether you're talking about pharmaceuticals or tobacco, recent studies "have all found that physicians with financial ties to manufacturers were significantly less likely to criticize the safety or efficacy of these agents." The bottom line . . . is the bottom line.

"Researchers with financial relationships with for-profit funders of research not surprisingly tend to overstate the favorableness of their own products and tend to be less likely to report unfavorable outcomes, especially issues surrounding safety or efficacy." Is there any reason to suspect that your corporation is any different?

Most of the "Supporting" Studies Were Inadequately Controlled

One of the favorite ways drug manufacturers design studies to skew results in favor of their product is to choose inappropriate controls. Just as a drug company might choose an inadequate dosing of the comparison drug to artificially inflate the results of its own product, many of the "supporting" studies of the Atkins Diet were compared to diets that were "low-fat" in name only— yet the Atkins Diet *still* failed to outperform them long-term.

In what was to become the single largest and longest controlled study of the Atkins Diet to date, researchers published "A low-carbohydrate as compared to a low-fat diet in severe obesity" in the *New England Journal of Medicine*. Both the press and the Atkins Corporation heralded the findings as proof that low-carb diets were in some ways superior to low-fat diets. The problem is that the control group was never actually on a low-fat diet. They started out eating 33% calories from fat like the rest of America, and at the end of the six-month study period in which they were supposedly switched to a "low-fat" diet, they were eating . . . 33% calories from fat.

At the end of a year, those who remained in the "low-fat" group were eating even more fat than average—34% calories from fat—yet you continued to erroneously describe this as a low-fat diet. On your website, "Atkins professionals" claim that the "low-fat" control group "followed a calorie-restricted diet with less than 30% of calories from fat per day." This is false. And even though the study was inadequately controlled, the low-carb diet, according to the researchers, "provided no weight loss advantage" compared to the group that hardly seemed to be on a diet at all.

This is the same story we see in every single year-long controlled trial of low-carb diets. Not a single one showed significantly more weight lost at the end of the year on the low-carb diets than on the control "low-fat" diets. And in the two yearlong studies that compared low-carb diets to actual low-fat diets, the low-fat diets seemed to win.

Most of the studies cited as "supporting Atkins" lasted at most a few months, half had 15 or fewer people on the diet, and a third lacked any control group at all. And the majority of those that did randomize people into a control group compared low-carb diets to "low-fat" diets containing between 29% and 35% calories from fat. That is not a low-fat diet.

Calorie-restricted, portion-controlled, moderate-fat (30%) diets have a consistent history of failure to maintain long-term weight loss. What better diet to assign to a comparison group, then, to increase the odds that low-carb diets will show more weight loss? And *still*, even using inadequate controls, low-carb diets failed to outperform control "low-fat" diets in every single long-term study ever done.

A diet truly low in fat (25% or less) plus exercise is the only approach found to provide long-term successful weight loss, based on a study of 5,000 Americans who lost an average of more than 70 pounds each and kept it off for more than six years. According to one of the chief investigators of that study, "Almost nobody's on a low-carbohydrate diet."

• **AtkinsFacts.org Relies on Outdated Critiques**

Furthermore, by devoting a significant portion of your critique to the first edition of Dr. Atkins' diet book, published in 1972,

you impart the misleading impression that Atkins has not incor-
porated the numerous advances in medical and nutritional
research (such as the recognition of lipid subclasses as risk fac-
tors for heart disease) that have since occurred.

First of all, most of the over 500 references I cite are from 2002 or later. Second, the official condemnations of the Atkins Diet from the medical authorities of the 1970s continue to hold weight to this day. According to your own website, the Atkins Corporation claims that that the basic tenets of the Atkins Diet have remained "consistent since 1972," insisting that "nothing in the earlier books is wrong." The medical authorities back then, and today, disagree.

- **AtkinsFacts.org Understates the Amount of Fiber in the Diet**

   In another instance, you report that the Induction Phase of
   the ANA [Atkins Diet] only provides two grams of fiber a
   day (page 13 [AtkinsExposed.org]). This number was not
   calculated by doing an independent nutrient analysis based
   on the menus provided in Atkins' New Diet Revolution, and
   although reference is made to the 1999 edition of the book,
   nowhere does the book mention that only two grams of fiber
   are provided. In fact, the Induction Phase using just whole
   foods would deliver approximately 18 grams of fiber per day.
   The addition of one Advantage bar includes an additional
   6–10 grams of fiber per day.

Although your letter repeatedly accuses AtkinsFacts.org of making false statements, you give almost no examples. The few examples you do offer are wrong. This accusation about fiber content is no exception.

Based on a nutritional analysis of *Dr. Atkins' New Diet Revolution* (M. Evans & Co., 1999), pp. 257–259, using Nutritionist V., Version 2.0, for Windows 98 (First DataBank, Inc., Hearst Corporation, San Bruno, CA), the fiber content of a "Typical Induction Menu" is 2 grams, exactly as I stated in the "Constipation" section.

You imply, though, that an "independent nutrient analysis" would find that "In fact, the Induction Phase . . . would deliver approximately 18 grams of fiber per day." There have been three such independent nutrient analyses done—one by Tufts University, another published in the *Journal of the American College of Nutrition*, and a third in the 2004 volume of the *Journal of the American College of Cardiology*. Did they find that "in fact" the Atkins Diet would "deliver 18 grams of fiber a day"?

All three of the published independent nutrient analyses of the Atkins Diet calculated 4 grams of fiber.

Four grams of fiber is only 13% of the *minimum* recommended by the American College of Gastroenterology, 16% of the Food and Drug Administration's Daily Value and between only 10.5% (for men) and 16% (for women) of the National Academy of Sciences' Institute of Medicine recommended daily intake. Either way, and by any legitimate recommendation, the induction phase of the Atkins Diet is seriously deficient in fiber.

• **AtkinsFacts.org Purports That Atkins Claims Supplements Are Necessary**

Cost of Supplements. The site mentions the cost of vitamins and manufactured foods purportedly necessary to be purchased from Atkins in order to adhere to the ANA [Atkins Diet] (page 19 [AtkinsExposed.org]). However, these products are recommended only to supplement a variety of whole foods, including meats, cheeses, fruits, vegetables, and whole grains. The ANA [Atkins Diet] guidelines meet the federal minimum fruits and vegetables recommendations, including in the Induction Phase.

In regard to your objection that AtkinsFacts.org describes supplements as necessary on your diet, I refer you to the latest and last edition of Dr. Atkins' book, a chapter entitled "Nutritional Supplements: Don't Even Think of Getting Along Without Them."

Also, as documented in the "Malnutrition" section, the Atkins Diet most certainly does not meet minimum federal recommendations for fruits and vegetables according to an independent peer-reviewed nutritional analysis published in the *Journal of the American College of Nutrition*. The Atkins Diet was found to provide fewer than three servings of fruits and vegetables per day, while current federal guidelines recommend at least five.

Atkins Implies That Their Diet Is Not Extraordinarily Constipating

Constipation can occur on any weight-loss program.

It is true that constipation can occur with any weight-loss program. However, even compared to other low-carb diets, the Atkins Diet is exemplary for its dearth of fiber. Compared to seven other popular diets, the Atkins Diet is by far the lowest in fiber.

Independent nutritional analyses have found that the initial phase of the Atkins Diet, to which dieters may have to repeatedly return, has less than 15% of the minimum daily requirement for fiber as recommended by the American College of Gastroenterology.

As documented in the Constipation section, one study funded by Atkins found that 70% of the patients on the Atkins Diet suffered from constipation. Dr. Atkins himself even admitted that nearly all of his patients were constipated.

- **AtkinsFacts.org Engages in Selective Citation**

  Cancer Risk. You selectively refer to articles to support your claim that the ANA [Atkins Diet] can increase the risk of cancer. Interestingly, this is something you accused Dr. Atkins of doing at page 6 of your site. In fact, studies you omit from your discussion contradict your conclusions.

To avoid any risk of selective citation, let me jump right to the most comprehensive report ever published on diet and cancer in history. The *AICR/WCRF Expert Report, Food, Nutrition and the Prevention of Cancer: A Global Perspective* took over four years to complete, reviewed 4,500 studies from thousands of researchers across the globe, and became a landmark scientific consensus document written by the top cancer researchers in the world. Their number one recommendation was, "Choose a diet that is predominantly plant-based, rich in a variety of fruits, vegetables, nuts, and beans with minimally processed starchy foods." In other words, essentially the opposite of the Atkins Diet.

The 2004 World Health Organization guidelines are consistent with the AICR/WCRF Expert Report in calling for limiting the consumption of saturated animal fats and "increasing the consumption of fruits, vegetables, legumes [beans, peas and lentils], whole grains, and nuts."

As documented in the Cancer section, it is no wonder the American Institute for Cancer Research and the American Cancer Society go out of their way to discourage low-carb diets.

Atkins Claims the Atkins Diet May Prevent Colon Cancer

You seem to disagree with the American Cancer Society's assessment. Dr. Atkins was asked, for example, if "a lot of red meat could cause colon cancer." He replied that there was "very little evidence to support the viewpoint." On your official web-site, an Atkins co-author even states that "a controlled-carbohydrate eating plan could be a valuable way to help prevent colorectal cancer."

Why then does the American Cancer Society say that "consumption of meat—especially red meats—has been linked to cancers at several sites, most notably colon and prostate?" Is the American Cancer Society merely omitting studies that "contradict" their conclusion?

So as to avoid the risk of selective citation, let me consult the latest reviews of the evidence. A review in 2002 concluded that a "preponderance" of evidence "suggests that minimizing red meat intake would result in decreased risk of this cancer [colorectal cancer]." According to a consensus statement by some of the top cancer researchers in the world, red meat consumption may be related to prostate cancer as well.

The only review since was published in 2004. Researchers at Harvard, Oxford, and the National Cancer Institute once again reviewed the available evidence and agreed that eating "a lot of red meat" probably does indeed increase one's risk for colon and rectal cancer.

Atkins Claims the Atkins Diet Could Prevent Breast Cancer Too

Your website also claims that "doing Atkins is the ideal way" to control breast cancer risk: "A controlled carb way of eating almost automatically lowers your risk of breast cancer." Eating over a half cup of lard's worth of saturated fat every day is an "ideal way" to prevent breast cancer?

Your website claims, "Saturated fat, the kind found in meat, butter, cheese and other animal foods as well as tropical oils, hasn't been shown to have any effect on your risk of breast cancer—whether positive or negative." To support this surprising claim, the Atkins website cites an article published in 1997 that, upon review, doesn't address the topic at all.

Although your website claims that "At Atkins Nutritionals we pride ourselves on bringing you the most accurate, well-researched information on every topic we cover," it seems that you are not, in fact, citing articles accurately.

The most comprehensive report ever published on diet and cancer in history, reviewing thousands of studies, concluded that diets high in saturated fat were linked to breast cancer. A re-review of the topic in 2003 came to the same conclusion. And September 2004 brought us yet another systematic meta-analysis of published studies that showed once again that saturated fat intake is indeed "associated with an increased risk of breast cancer."

Atkins Ignores Trans Fats in the Atkins Diet

Dr. Atkins was asked, "Isn't the consumption of fat related to cancer?" He replied, "According to the multitude of studies published, fat per se was not linked to cancer, with the exception of trans fats, which are not included in the Atkins Nutritional Approach." This is incorrect on two counts. First of all, trans fats are not the only exception; saturated animal fat has been linked to cancers of the breast, prostate, endometrium, lung, and pancreas. And second, trans fats *are* included throughout the Atkins Diet.

In nature, trans fats are found mainly in animal fat. The food industry, however, found a way to synthetically create these toxic fats by hardening vegetable oil in a process called hydrogenation, which rearranges atoms to make them behave more like animal fats. Although most of America's trans-fat intake comes from processed foods containing partially hydrogenated oils, a fifth of the trans fats American adults consume comes from animal products.

According to the official National Nutrient Database, 5% of the fat in a burger is trans fat. The fat in cheese averages 3% trans fat, and butter can be up to 7% trans fat. Hot-dog and turkey fat average about 4% trans fats, and the fat in pork rinds is 1% trans fat.

Is 1% a problem, though? The most prestigious scientific body in the United States, the National Academy of Science, concluded that the only safe intake of trans fat is zero. In their report condemning trans fats they couldn't even assign a Tolerable Upper Daily Limit of intake because "any incremental increase in trans fatty acid intake increases coronary heart disease risk."

Trans fats, according to the report, "are unavoidable on ordinary, non-vegan diets. . . ." One of the authors of the report, a nutritional epidemiologist at the Harvard School of Public Health, explained why they didn't recommend a vegan diet: "We can't tell people to stop eating all meat and all dairy products," he said. "Well, we could tell people to become vegetarians," he added. "If we were truly basing this only on science, we would, but it is a bit extreme."

"Nevertheless," the report concludes, "it is recommended that trans fatty acid consumption be as low as possible while consuming a nutritionally adequate diet." The Atkins Diet seems to accomplish neither.

Incidentally, the Atkins director of education and research is convinced that "Researchers at Harvard and elsewhere have made it plain that trans fatty acids have been a killer since the 1930s. . . ." Yet the 1972 *Dr. Atkins' Diet Revolution* recommended "unlimited" quantities of vegetable shortening, the single most concentrated source of trans fatty acids in the food supply. Though the dangers of trans fats had been known "since the 1930s," it took Atkins, who is painted as a "pioneer" and an "innovator," until the 1980s before he finally took a position against them.

Atkins' "Best Evidence" Contradicts Corporation's Position

"Does a high-fat diet cause breast cancer?" Your website

responds: "Just the opposite—the right kinds of dietary fat may help prevent it. The best evidence for this comes from Harvard's ongoing Nurses' Health Study. In 1992 this long-running study of more than 100,000 women showed no connection between the amount or type of dietary fat the subjects ate and their risk of getting breast cancer."

I agree that the Harvard Nurses' Health Studies represent the best evidence. It was, in fact, those very studies that showed in 2003 that young women with the highest intake of red meat and butterfat had over a 75% greater risk of developing breast cancer.

It's true that total fat consumption has not been convincingly linked to cancer risk, but this is because researchers weren't taking into account the difference between animal fats and vegetable fats. There is evidence that some types of plant fat, like olive oil, may protect against breast cancer. So there are indeed "right kinds of dietary fat," but the saturated fat pushed by Atkins is the wrong kind.

In the Nurses' Health Study that followed nearly 100,000 premenopausal women, Harvard researchers separated out the animal fat and found that pre-menopausal women who consumed the most saturated animal fat had a significantly greater chance of developing breast cancer. They concluded, "Intake of animal fat, mainly from red meat and high-fat dairy foods, during premenopausal years is associated with an increased risk of breast cancer."

In a University of Cambridge study published the same week, researchers found that women reportedly eating 34 grams of saturated fat a day seemed to roughly double their breast cancer risk compared to women who ate only 11 grams of saturated fat. Followers of your diet, as reported in a "Research Supporting Atkins" study on your website, eat as many as 67 grams of saturated fat a day.

Atkins Claims No Excess Protein-Cancer Link

Dr. Atkins was asked "What is the relationship between excessive protein consumption and cancer?" He replied, "No one has ever demonstrated a relationship between excessive protein consumption and cancer."

Once again, this is incorrect. Protein intake, particularly animal protein intake, has been linked to brain tumors, breast cancer, pancreatic cancer, stomach cancer, endometrial cancer, kidney cancer, laryngeal cancer, esophageal cancer—even lung cancer. Excess animal protein has also been deemed an " 'aggressive' risk factor for colon cancer."

Atkins Misrepresents Data Presented at a Conference

One of the questions addressed in the "Frequently Asked Questions" section of your website is "Doesn't a high-fat diet increase cancer risk?" In your answer, you argue that there is no link between meat and colon cancer, and base your argument solely on preliminary, unpublished data from a single investigation described at a meeting that took place years ago. Further, even that data was misrepresented.

The meeting was the European Conference on Nutrition and Cancer back in 2001, where the preliminary findings of the European Prospective Investigation into Cancer (EPIC) were presented. You claim that the findings "raised questions about the long-held belief that eating red meat or other animal-based foods can increase the risk of cancer."

I decided to look at the official account of that conference published by the World Health Organization in order to respond to your claims.

Dr. Atkins said that "The European conference that studied the lifestyles of more than 500,000 individuals confirmed that there is not link [sic] between meat consumption and increased risk of colon and rectal cancer." To clarify, the population studied numbered 472,000, and this is what the researchers actually said: "The meat-colorectal cancer association has been investigated by at least 34 case-control and 14 cohort studies, which collected information on various types of meat products. The overall results suggest that frequent consumption of red meat, mainly beef, veal, pork and lamb, is associated with a 20–40% increase in colorectal cancer risk. . . ."

True, the increase in colorectal cancer risk associated with red meat in the "very preliminary" data from the EPIC study were "for the moment" not statistically significant, but, as the investigators note, "As the follow-up is in progress, these first results should be interpreted with caution." This is what Atkins claimed "confirmed" that there was no link, even though the very source he cited mentions almost 50 studies whose "overall results" show that there is a link. Therefore, the source you cite to support your claim in fact refutes it.

According to the study's coordinator, chief of the nutrition division at the International Agency for Research on Cancer, those eating just 2 ounces of processed meat (like bacon or ham) a day had a 50% greater risk of developing cancer of the colon or rectum. Two ounces is just one jumbo hot dog.

An independent review given at that same conference concluded, "High intakes of red meat, and particularly of processed meat, are associated with a moderate but significant increase in colorectal cancer risk and suggest that colorectal cancer incidence could be decreased by reducing red and processed meat intakes in populations where intake is high." This is in agreement with a 2004 review published by one of the lead EPIC study investigators.

Other independent research provided at the conference— that you argue challenges the "long-held misconceptions about . . . animal products"—found that those eating more than 5.5

grams of fatty red meat a day (roughly a single teaspoon of ground beef) seemed to have over twice the risk of developing colon or rectal cancer. In an article entitled "Red meat could be as carcinogenic as tobacco," Associated Press writer Emma Ross noted that new research presented at the conference indicated that eating red meat could raise the level of certain colon carcinogens as much as smoking does.

According to the official account, what the EPIC study did show was that fruit consumption seemed to significantly protect against colon and rectal cancer and the more fiber people ate, the lower their risk. Those eating just 25 grams of fiber a day seemed to cut their risk by about 40%.

Fruit consumption alone seems to protect one from numerous cancers and may reduce heart disease mortality, cancer and total mortality. However, Dr. Atkins warned readers that, even during later, more liberal phases of his diet, eating fruit will "always" be "somewhat risky"—when in fact the reverse may be true.

- **AtkinsFact.org Makes "Unsupported" Arguments About Bone Risk**

Your arguments . . . that the ANA [Atkins Diet] can adversely affect bones and kidney function are similarly unsupported. Urinary calcium loss is not an inevitable result of a low-carbohydrate dietary regimen.

This claim is similar to the one made in "Talking About Atkins to Your Doctor," a section of your website that explains that "you may have to educate your health-care provider a bit about exactly what's involved with Atkins." If, for example, one's doctor is concerned that eating too much meat may leach calcium from one's bones, you recommend telling the doctor, "This is another myth that has been disproved." Before confronting their doctors, though, dieters may want to know the whole story.

The truth is that we've known for 80 years that high protein intake, particularly the protein found in beef, fish, and chicken, increases calcium loss through the urine.

In 2002, the World Health Organization and the Food and Agriculture Organization of the United Nations published the long-awaited report *Human Vitamin and Mineral Requirements*. They concluded that animal protein intake has a "major effect" on calcium requirements. Using an equation based on over 200 calcium balance studies, they calculate that those who eat 60 grams of animal protein lose the equivalent of hundreds of milligrams of consumed calcium every day. Meanwhile, independent nutritional analyses find Atkins followers eating as much as *140* grams of animal protein a day.

For documentation of what this kind of acid load might do to one's bones, see the section "Peeing Your Bones Down the Toilet."

Atkins Ignores the Studies That Actually Measure Fracture Risk

Although some short-term studies reveal a net urinary calcium loss, long-term studies directly examining bone loss via DEXA scan (a superior indicator of bone health relative to urinary calcium) reveal no bone loss.

It is evident that you focus on risk indicators rather than disease endpoints. Your website, for example, discusses cardiac risk factors without referencing the one study that actually measured blood flow in the hearts of Atkins dieters and in fact showed a significant worsening of their heart disease. Although DEXA scans may be superior to urinary calcium measurements, arguably the best indicator would be assessing a person's risk of actually suffering a bone fracture. The Harvard Nurses' Health Study, which followed over 85,000 nurses for a dozen years, found that those eating just a serving of red meat a day had a significantly increased fracture risk.

While plant-based proteins did not show a deleterious effect, women in the Nurses' Study eating more animal protein had a significantly increased risk of forearm fracture. Another study, which followed a thousand women, linked meat consumption to hip fracture risk as well. The investigators concluded, "This suggests that an increase in vegetable protein intake and a decrease in animal protein intake may decrease bone loss and the risk of hip fracture." The only other study that looked at a large group of the general population over time found that those consuming as much meat and egg protein and as little calcium as do Atkins dieters *doubled* their risk of hip fracture.

Your website lists 15 "selected" studies, though, that claim to show that the Atkins Diet doesn't adversely affect calcium and bone metabolism. Many of the conflicting results are based on what's called the "biphasic" effect of protein on bone health. Too much protein can increase fracture risk, but too little protein can as well, since protein makes up about 50% of bone tissue. So some studies involving elderly subjects who may have been suffering from "protein undernutrition" have shown less bone loss or fracture risk with higher protein intakes, but low protein intake alone may be a marker of frailty or poor nutritional status in general. In fact, studies show that protein malnutrition in the elderly may increase hip fracture rate just by increasing their propensity to fall.

Studies not restricted to the elderly, though, have more clearly found that those who eat the most animal protein may be putting their bones at risk.

Atkins Falsely Claims Followers Are Getting Enough Calcium

Atkins offers a variety of foods rich in calcium in all phases of the program, including Induction. . . .

Animal protein causes calcium loss, but studies have shown that if one consumes enough calcium, one may be able to mediate the effects of that protein. The problem is that the Atkins Diet can also be seriously deficient in calcium. The Atkins "Debunking the Myths" webpage, though, calls such a charge just another "fallacy," claiming that "While you're doing Atkins you will get 100% of the Recommended Daily Intake of calcium. . . ."

According to independent nutritional analyses, this is incorrect. The estimated calcium content of the Atkins Diet during Induction, according to one analysis, is 373 mg, less than 40% of the Recommended Daily Intake. Tufts calls the low calcium content of the Atkins Diet (even after Induction) one of its "serious dietary shortfalls."

• **AtkinsFacts.org Spreads "the Biggest Myth of All" About Kidney Risk**

Nor does the ANA [Atkins Diet] adversely affect kidney function. Although Atkins recommends that individuals with renal impairment seek medical approval from their personal physician prior to starting the ANA [Atkins Diet], studies have shown that high protein intake was not associated with renal function decline in women with normal renal function.

According to your website, the fact that Atkins followers risk kidney damage "may be the biggest myth of all." You counter this "fallacy" that eating too much protein on the Atkins Diet is bad for one's kidneys with "Fact: Too many people believe this untruth simply because it has been repeated so often that even intelligent health professionals assume it must have been reported somewhere. But the fact is that it has never been reported anywhere. No one has as yet produced a study for review, or even cite a specific case in which a diet high in protein causes any form of kidney disorder." Again, this is simply incorrect.

Atkins Dismisses the Harvard Nurses' Study's Conclusions

You dismiss the Harvard Nurses' Study's finding that high meat protein intake may worsen kidney function in part because the diet of the women in the study was "not a low-carbohydrate diet analogous to the ANA [Atkins Diet]." This is true. The "excessive" amount of protein that furthered kidney damage in the women in the Nurses' Study is only about half of what one might expect to get on the Atkins Diet. Please see the "Kidney Damage" section of this book for more about kidney risk.

Atkins Claims Diet is High-Fat, Not High-Protein

You claim your diet is not an "excessively high-protein regimen." The Atkins Diet, you argue, "should be more appropriately be called a high-fat regimen." It is both. Even according to one of the "Research Supporting Atkins" studies, followers of the Atkins Diet eat as much as 156 grams of protein a day, over 250% of what most people need.

- **AtkinsFacts.org Objectionably Asserts Diet Is Bad for Heart**

    You assert . . . that the ANA adversely affects the lipid profile, thereby increasing risk of cardiovascular disease. However, in the studies referenced by Atkins at

http://atkins.com/science/researchsupportingatkins.html,
the majority of subjects following a low-carbohydrate diet
experience favorable responses (e.g., a decrease in serum
triglycerides or LDL and an increase in serum HDL)
(Westman 2002).

Atkins Ignores Proof That the Atkins Diet Clogs Arteries

Based on one analysis of your diet published in the *American Journal of Clinical Nutrition*, long-term use of the Atkins Diet is expected to raise coronary heart disease risk by over 50%. But before one even addresses the question of risk factors, as documented in "The Proof Is in the SPECT Scan," there was a study published in the peer-reviewed medical literature that actually measured what was happening to people's arteries on the Atkins Diet. The results, posted online, validate the claim that the Atkins Diet, according to the American Dietetic Association, is "a heart attack waiting to happen."

Atkins Exaggerates the Benefit of Lowering Triglycerides

Yes, the Atkins Diet can consistently reduce triglyceride levels, but even according to your own researchers, the same cannot be said for the most important risk factor, LDL cholesterol. This may be why after just months on your diet, people's arteries have been shown to clog so rapidly. Your claim that triglycerides are as big a threat to heart health as cholesterol—or even bigger—is demonstrably false.

Every leading authority—the American Dietetic, Diabetes, Heart, Hospital, Nurses, Public Health and Medical Associations, the American Colleges of Cardiology, Nutrition and Preventive Medicine—all agree that LDL cholesterol is the single most important target for preventing heart disease.

The National Heart, Lung, and Blood Institute coordinates a coalition of more than 40 major medical and health associations, community programs, and governmental agencies whose 27-member Expert Panel took nearly two years to develop the latest guidelines for the prevention of heart disease. "For all persons with borderline high or high triglycerides," the guidelines state, "the primary aim of therapy is to achieve the target goal for LDL cholesterol."

Elevated triglycerides may not even be an independent risk factor for heart disease. "There are little data," concludes one review, "that triglyceride reduction improves cardiovascular event rate." This is why the Expert Panel concentrates on lowering LDL cholesterol levels, an intervention proven to extend life and lower the risk of heart attacks.

Atkins Distorts the Record on Cholesterol

A rise in serum LDL levels is not an inevitable response to low-carbohydrate dietary regimens. Some studies report no statistically significant changes in LDL levels (Stern, 2004; Yancy, 2004) or a statistically significant reduction (Westman, 2002) in LDL levels.

As documented in the section "Atkins Distorted His Record on Cholesterol" [AtkinsExposed.org], the Atkins Diet has failed to consistently improve the single most important risk factor for heart disease, LDL, or "bad" cholesterol. Your website, however, claims, "Almost every Atkins follower sees a drop in LDL ('bad') cholesterol." Even Atkins-funded researchers concede that this is incorrect. "Although the data is limited," they write, "very-low-carbohydrate diets tend to result in moderate increases in low-density lipoprotein [LDL] cholesterol. . . ."

Atkins Argues That Size Matters

Furthermore, some studies reveal that in subjects who experienced an increase in serum LDL levels, the increase is due

> to a greater number of large LDL particles (pattern A) and
> not an increase of atherogenic small LDL particles (pattern
> B) (Sharman 2004, Hays 2003, Sharman 2002). In addi-
> tion, in some instances, the opposite trend may occur in low-
> fat diets: "Paradoxically, a low-fat/high-carbohydrate diet
> exacerbates atherogenic dyslipidemia if the patient does not
> lose a significant amount of weight or increase his or her
> level of physical activity." (Volek 2002)

You admit that bad cholesterol may rise on your diet, but
argue that the rise may be mostly in *large* bad cholesterol (pattern "A") not the "atherogenic small" bad cholesterol (pattern
"B"). While earlier research done on rabbits indeed showed that
small LDL particles seemed more likely to infiltrate rabbit arteries, studies since then on the arteries of actual human beings
found that size doesn't matter.

Frank M. Sacks, M.D., professor of cardiovascular disease
prevention at Harvard, with over a hundred publications to his
name, reviewed all of the evidence surrounding LDL size in
2003. He found that some studies showed that in fact larger LDL
(the type that the Atkins Diet elevates) seemed more dangerous.
"Thus," he wrote, "large and small LDL are atherogenic, and it is
not possible to judge which if any is more harmful, overall."
Cleveland Clinic Medical Director (and vice president of the
American College of Cardiology) Steven Nissen, M.D., agrees
that LDL particle size simply isn't clinically useful.

"In summary," Dr. Sacks wrote, "the picture is emerging . . .
that small LDL does not have a special relationship to coronary
heart disease beyond its contribution to LDL concentration." He
concludes that "all LDL types should be viewed as harmful." In
other words, large or small, bad cholesterol is bad cholesterol.

True, if one switches to a low-fat diet centered around refined
sugars and starches one can suffer a relative increase in small

LDL particle and triglycerides. But low-fat diets based on whole foods can not only reduce the number of small LDL cholesterol particles (and triglyceride levels), but routinely drastically improve LDL cholesterol levels overall. Your diet does not allow for this, which may be why the arterial blockages in the hearts of your followers have been shown to worsen so dramatically.

Atkins Offers No Viable Alternative to Drugs

Dr. Atkins warned about the dangers associated with the cholesterol-lowering "statin" drugs, but his diet won't lower cholesterol enough to help dieters avoid a lifetime of these costly medications. On the contrary, the Atkins Diet has in fact been shown to seriously worsen heart disease.

Atkins claims that the National Heart, Lung, and Blood Institute Expert Panel that sets heart disease prevention guidelines advocates drugs as the "first line of defense." This is incorrect. The panel advocates "lifestyle changes as first-line therapy" and "the foundation" of prevention, and drugs typically only if lifestyle changes fail. The primary lifestyle change they recommend is "reduced intakes of saturated fat and cholesterol," exactly the opposite of what your diet can offer.

When it comes to diet, LDL cholesterol is the single most important risk factor for heart disease and the number one killer in the United States for both men and women. The immediate goal is to get one's LDL down to double digits, levels in fact seen in most people around the world. In Asia, for example, where low-fat diets are the norm and rates of heart disease are a fraction of those in Western countries, the average LDL of the entire population of 4 billion people is lower than 95. Although there is evidence that LDL levels between 50 and 70 may be ideal, an LDL level below 100 mg/dl "is now considered optimal for all individuals."

According to the editor-in-chief of the *American Journal of Cardiology*, the only two groups in America that seem to consistently reach that goal are those on cholesterol-lowering medications and those on a "pure vegetarian" diet. The only diet that seems to routinely bring one's bad cholesterol down into the target zone is one devoid of all saturated animal fat and cholesterol.

Based on the best current published data, the average LDL cholesterol level of Americans is estimated at 130 mg/dl. Studies show that the average LDL of healthy meat eaters (typically well-educated, lean non-smokers with high exercise levels) is 121, for those who just eat fish, 114; vegetarians almost make the mark at 106, and vegans seem the only dietary group that achieves the target LDL at 90 mg/dl.

While almost every single study of low-carb diets showed no reduction—or even an elevation—in LDL levels, the single uncontrolled Atkins-funded study you cite that showed a significant drop in LDL levels took six months to bring LDL levels from 136 to 126, numbers still very much in the danger zone.

For Americans to drop from 130 to under 100, they need at least a 23% drop in LDL. That's exactly how much a low-fat, primarily vegetarian diet can decrease LDL in three weeks based on a study of 4,587 adults. Compare that to the best that your dieters have been shown to achieve—a 7% drop in six months.

Cholesterol-lowering diets don't have to be low-fat, however. A full-fat, phytonutrient-rich vegan diet has been shown to lower LDL by 30% in two weeks—which is as much as one gets with cholesterol-lowering medications.

This may be the reason why, when researchers are able to directly measure the arterial blockages in the heart, vegetarian diets have been shown to reverse heart disease, increasing blood flow up to 40%, whereas those on your diet suffered a worsening of their blockages, *decreasing* blood flow 40%.

Atkins Exaggerates the Benefit of Raising HDL Cholesterol

Saturated fat can raise HDL (Hickey 2003, Westman 2002).

High HDL levels have shown to be protective against coronary heart disease. Therefore, even if LDL is slightly increased, the LDL/HDL ratio and total cholesterol/HDL ratio are still improved after following a low-carbohydrate, high-saturated-fat diet (Volek 2003).

This claim is similar to the one on your website that low HDL is a more important risk factor than elevated LDL. This is demonstrably false.

The Expert Panel that writes the federal U.S. heart disease prevention guidelines, representing a coalition of over 30 major medical organizations, could not even find "sufficient evidence to make HDL a target of treatment." They felt the centerpiece of the guidelines, aggressive lowering of the "bad cholesterol" LDL, should negate any increased risk associated with low "good cholesterol" HDL levels. "Thus, ATPIII [the Expert Panel] recommends that the first step in treating patients who are found to have a low HDL level is to lower the LDL level to goal," something the Atkins Diet can't do.

"Whether raising HDL per se will reduce risk for coronary heart disease," the panel concludes, "has not been resolved. . . . In all persons with low HDL cholesterol, the primary therapy is [to lower] LDL cholesterol."

The available evidence shows that the most important number is not HDL, not total cholesterol, not triglycerides, and not the size of the LDL particles, but the amount of LDL you have in your blood, the amount of this "bad" cholesterol you have circulating in your arteries. The Expert Panel recognized that high triglycerides, small LDL particles, and low HDL cholesterol are a "secondary target of risk-reduction therapy," but only "after the primary target—LDL cholesterol."

Significantly lowering one's LDL is more important than significantly raising one's HDL, though the studies done on low-carb diets typically show neither. It should come as no surprise, then, that in the only study to directly measure the effects of the Atkins Diet on the heart, the diet was shown to seriously weaken coronary artery blood flow to the heart.

Atkins Ignores "More Important" Risk Factors That Worsen on Atkins

According to your website, "Dr. Atkins does not believe that cholesterol elevations are as important a risk factor as . . . homocysteine and C-reactive protein." It is interesting to note, then, that even research he funded shows that both of these risk factors worsen on the Atkins Diet.

Homocysteine

"A byproduct of defective protein metabolism," one can read on your website, "elevated homocysteine levels are a powerful marker of heart disease and stroke risk." Homocysteine has also been linked to birth defects, fatal blood clots, depression, osteoporosis, and Alzheimer's Disease.

One can also read on your website that "The Atkins Nutritional Approach, in fact, is ideal for moderating homocysteine levels. . . ." No studies are offered to support this, but of the 34 studies you cite as "supporting" the Atkins Diet, only one study measured homocysteine levels, and in that study Atkins followers suffered a highly significant *worsening* of their homocysteine levels.

The American Heart Association has recommended a homocysteine level *under* 10 (mcmol/L). The Atkins website agrees: "Above 10 mcmol/L indicates an increasing risk of cardiovascular disease. . . ." Atkins notes that high homocysteine may also be related to cancer.

So what happened to people put on your diet? In just six weeks, their homocysteine levels rose from 9.5 to 10.6. In their conclusion, the researchers deemed this elevation "concerning."

In the yearlong study that compared your diet to a vegan diet, homocysteine levels again tended to rise on the Atkins Diet and fall on the vegan diet. A *Preventive Medicine* article entitled "Vegan diet-based lifestyle program rapidly lowers homocysteine levels" stated that after just one week on a vegan diet, those with elevated homocysteine levels experienced a drop from an average of 11.3 down to 9.2, a highly significant drop of 19% in just a single week.

Homocysteine, a neurotoxic and vasculotoxic compound linked to dementia, miscarriages, and stroke, and which Atkins himself deemed a more important risk factor than cholesterol, became further elevated in both of the two studies that measured homocysteine levels on the Atkins Diet.

C-Reactive Protein

Atkins also felt that C-reactive protein (CRP) was a more important risk factor than elevated cholesterol levels. "Chronically inflamed blood vessels are widely regarded as part of the atherosclerotic disease process," reads your website. "Research has found that high levels of . . . C-reactive protein, a marker of inflammation, increased the risk of heart disease by four and one-half times." C-reactive protein has been associated with stroke risk as well.

Like LDL cholesterol, simply losing weight *should* lower your CRP levels. How much CRP you have circulating in your blood has been found to be "strictly related to body fatness." Yet every single published study "supporting" Atkins showed that the Atkins Diet was ineffective in lowering CRP. In fact, one of them showed that after just six weeks on the Atkins Diet CRP levels tended to more than double despite a loss of body fat.

One unpublished meeting abstract on your website did show a decrease in CRP levels on the Atkins Diet, but two others did not. The year-long study that compared your diet to the Ornish

Diet, Weight Watchers and the Zone Diet found that C-reactive protein levels were significantly lowered by the Ornish Diet and by Weight Watchers, but not by the Atkins Diet.

Just two weeks on a low-fat, primarily vegetarian diet with exercise, however, can lower CRP levels 45%. Two weeks on a phytonutrient-rich, full-fat vegan diet with no additional exercise dropped CRP levels an average of 30%, as much as one sees with the use of statin drugs. Meanwhile, your diet evidently causes so much inflammation within the body that CRP levels don't seem to drop at all despite significant weight loss.

Fibrinogen, another inflammatory risk factor associated with heart attack and stroke risk, tends to rise on the Atkins Diet and drop on control low-fat diets. The same thing happens with Lp(a).

If LDL is to be considered bad cholesterol, Lp(a) is *really* bad cholesterol. The Atkins website agrees that Lp(a) is a "strong risk factor for heart disease and stroke." It also tends to rise on the Atkins Diet and fall on the control vegan diet.

Even taking into account some of the cardiac risk factors deemed most important by Atkins, the available evidence clearly demonstrates that the Atkins Diet may dramatically increase one's risk for heart disease.

- **AtkinsFacts.org Makes "Misleading" Assertion About Saturated Fat**

  Your assertions at page 26 [AtkinsExposed.org] regarding the health effects of saturated fats are misleading. Studies looking at the effects of saturated fat on LDL and total cholesterol have primarily been conducted in conjunction with a high-carbohydrate diet.

Similarly, from your website: "Is it OK for me to consume more than 20% of my calories in the form of saturated fat?

Absolutely," you replied, "you're fine as long as you're also follow-ing the rules of the ANA [Atkins Diet], which include controlling your carbs." Dr. Frank M. Sacks, a professor of cardiovascular disease prevention at the Harvard School of Public Health, called this argument simply "ridiculous."

As documented in the section "Saturated Fat and Cholesterol Are Bad for You" [AtkinsExposed.org], the balance of evidence clearly shows that intake of saturated animal fat is associated with increased risk of cancer, diabetes, and heart disease. "I still don't understand the [Atkins] rationale in limiting trans fats and not saturated fat," said a spokesperson for the American Dietetic Association and director of Nutrition Therapy at the Cleveland Clinic Foundation. "Trans fats act very similarly in the body as saturated fat—they both increase LDL 'bad' cholesterol. . . ."

The best dietary strategy for reducing one's risk of dying from the number one killer in the United States is to reduce one's con-sumption of saturated fat and cholesterol. The evidence backing this, according to the American Heart Association, is "overwhelm-ing." A 2004 review of the evidence agreed, and recommended less than 7% of daily calories from saturated fat. Followers of your diet, as reported in a "Research Supporting Atkins" study, eat as much as 30% of their calories from saturated fat.

Atkins Corporation Mislabels and Then Misrepresents Studies

Your website claims "saturated fats aren't bad." According to Colette Heimowitz, M.S., the Atkins director of education and research, saturated fat has a "heart-healthy role. . . . In fact," she writes, "some large epidemiological trials, including the well-known Framingham Nurses' Study, have shown no correlation between saturated fat and heart disease, stroke, or breast cancer. In fact, the more saturated fat and cholesterol participants con-sumed, the lower their risk of heart disease."

There is no such thing as the "well-known Framingham Nurses' Study." Ms. Heimowitz must be thinking of either the Framingham Heart Study or the Harvard Nurses' Health Study. In either case, she is mistaken.

The Atkins director presumably wasn't talking about the Harvard Nurses' Study, as it showed specifically that the saturated fat found in Atkins favorites like beef, pork, lamb, cheese, butter, and lard was associated with greater risk of coronary heart disease. She must have been referring to the Framingham Heart study.

In a section of the Atkins website entitled "Debunking the Myths" you "debunk" the "fallacy" that "a liberal intake of high-fat meats . . . will raise cholesterol levels, ultimately leading to heart disease." The "fact," you claim, is that, according to the famous Framingham Heart Study, consuming less fat and cholesterol leads to higher blood cholesterol.

In its 56-year history, the Framingham Heart Study produced over 1,000 scientific papers. So as to not misrepresent any part of this important study, let me defer to Dr. William Castelli, who directed the Framingham Heart Study for over 26 years and is currently the director of the Framingham Cardiovascular Center.

Dr. Castelli was asked to directly respond to these claims. This is what he said: "That quote is correct but its interpretation by Atkins and Sugar Busters and others is wrong. The data are diet history data. Very weak science!!! . . . Better science, where I lock you up in a metabolic ward, has taught us that lowering the saturated fat, the cholesterol in the diet lowers cholesterol. Even better, over a dozen diet trials in the history of medicine which took people off the high-fat diet lowered their cholesterols and 4–5 years out they lowered their heart attack rate. Has Atkins or Sugar Busters shown that they lower the heart attack rate?"

"If Americans adopted a vegetarian diet," Castelli says of the heart disease epidemic, "the whole thing [heart attack risk] would disappear."

Atkins Implies the Type of Saturated Fat in Beef Is Benign

In "The Truth About Fat" your website argues that it is "absolutely" OK to consume more than 20% of calories in one's diet from saturated fat. "In fact," the article reads, "one-third of the fat in beef is stearic acid, which has been found to have a neutral or cholesterol-lowering effect." This is a classic deceptive tactic used by the chocolate industry.

If you go to a typical candy manufacturer's website, you can learn that indeed chocolate isn't bad for you because the predominant saturated fat, stearic acid, has a "neutral effect on blood cholesterol levels." Hershey's corporate website and that of the Mars candy bar corporation agree. So does the beef industry.

Even if stearic acid were benign, beef and chocolate also have other saturated fats, like lauric and myristic fatty acids, that do raise one's bad cholesterol and have been strongly linked with early heart attack. And stearic acid is far from benign. In fact, in the Harvard Nurses' Study, which followed over 80,000 women for over a decade, stearic acid was found to increase the risk of coronary heart disease even more than other saturated fats.

Though stearic acid may not affect cholesterol levels, its ability to thicken the blood and predispose it to clotting may be why it has been shown to be so pathogenic.

Please be advised that if you persist in misrepresenting the Atkins Nutritional Approach and the research supporting the ANA, [Atkins Diet] you do so at your own risk. We intend to monitor closely the AtkinsFacts.org website and other oral and written statements by you.

I intend to continue to warn the public about the serious potential dangers your diet presents. "When unproven science becomes a sales pitch," declared a spokesperson for the American Institute for Cancer Research about low-carb diets, "some people get rich and the rest of us get ripped off."

MICHAEL GREGER, MD

REFERENCES

Introduction

ix   *broke publishing records*: Martin D. "Dr. Robert C. Atkins, author of contro-versial but best-selling diet books, is dead at 72." *The New York Times* 18 April 2003:D9.

ix   *dozens of print*: Stewart DL. "Thin memories—Dr. Atkins: Author of contro-versial diet has Dayton roots, but his heart's in NYC." *Dayton Daily News* 20 February 2002.

ix   *all across the country*: Howard P and S Treadwell. "Dr. Atkins says he's sorry." *The New York Weekly* 26 March 1973.
<http://www.AtkinsExposed.org/atkins/117/Partnership_for_Essential_Nutri-tion.htm>.

ix   *serious threat to health*: U.S. Senate Select Committee on Nutrition and Human Needs. "Obesity and fad diets." 12 April 1973:CIS S581-13.

ix   *dangerous nonsense*: Ibid.

ix   *Of all the bizarre*: Smith BB. "Doctor sheds two chins—by eliminating carbo-hydrates." *Houston Chronicle* 9 March 1973.

ix   *$5 million lawsuit*: "Diet doctor threatens suit." Associated Press 11 June 1981.

x   *radiation-induced leukemia*: Kurzweil R. *The 10% Solution for a Healthy Life.* Three Rivers Press (CA), 1995.

x   *continued his lawsuit*: Lovendale M. "The Pritikin-Atkins debate (1979): Introduction and the science of nutrition."
<http://www.preventivecare.com/media.htm>.

x   *autopsy findings were published*: Hubbard JD, Inkeles S, and RJ Barnard. "Nathan Pritikin's heart." *New England Journal of Medicine* 313(1985):52.

x   *medical examiner's report*: "The Atkins empire strikes back." Scripps Howard News Service 19 February 2004.
<http://www.fumento.com/fat/empire.html>.

x   *extraordinarily healthy cardiovascular system*: Atkins Nutritionals, Inc. "State-ment on the status of Dr. Robert C. Atkins' health from Dr. Atkins and from the chief executive officer/president of the Atkins Companies." News release 25 April 2002.

x   *boasted to Katie Couric*: Sulmers C and C Campbell. "The diet martyr." *New York Magazine* 15 March 2004.

x   *30 to 40% blocked*: Ibid.

x   *on* Larry King Live: Interview with Veronica Atkins. *Larry King Live.* CNN. 16 February 2004.

xi   *new blockage*: Atkins V. "Statement by Veronica Atkins on the illegal distribu-
     tion of personal medical information regarding her late husband, Dr. Robert
     C. Atkins." April 2004.
     <http://atkins.com/about/recentnews/wsjresponse.html>.
xi   *Atkins wasn't being straightforward*: Borger G. "Dr. Bernadine Healy of *US
     News and World Report* discusses Dr. Robert Atkins' medical history and diet."
     CNBC News Transcripts. *Capital Report* 10 February 2004.
xi   *risk their health*: St Jeor ST, et al. Nutrition Committee of the Council on
     Nutrition, Physical Activity, and Metabolism of the American Heart Associa-
     tion. "Dietary protein and weight reduction: A statement for healthcare pro-
     fessionals from the Nutrition Committee of the Council on Nutrition,
     Physical Activity, and Metabolism of the American Heart Association." *Circu-
     lation* 104(2001):1869–74.
xi   *1,864 new "low-carb"*: Adamy J. "Some food makers trim low-carb plans as
     trend slows." *Wall Street Journal* 12 July 2004:B1.
xi   *low-carb gummy bears*: "U.S. candy makers slim down their treats." *Aging and
     Elder Health Week* 4 July 2004:45.
xi   *Hershey's*: Reitman V. "Coming soon: low-carb potatoes; long spurned by
     Atkins dieters, the less-starchy spud is poised for a comeback next year." *Los
     Angeles Times* 2 August 2004:F8.
xi   *Nestle*: Marsh S and J Bale. "Low fat is old hat as supermarkets rush to feed
     growing appetite for Atkins." *The Times* (London) 2 August 2004:7.
xi   *reduced-carb version*: Matthews S. "Low-carb trend may be peaking as Kellogg
     CEO sees product glut." *Chicago Sun-Times* 27 July 2004:56.
xi   *lower-carb doughnut*: Bhatnager P. "Low-carb bubble about to burst?"
     CNN/Money 22 March 2004.
xi   *hog prices*: Vansickle J. "Hog prices, demand soar." *National Hog Farmer* 15
     July 2004.
xi   *experts very concerned*: Partnership for Essential Nutrition. "Low-carbohydrate
     diets: Do they work and are they healthy?"
     <http://www.essentialnutrition.org/lowcarb.php>.
xi   *consistent since 1972*: Atkins Nutritionals, Inc. "Atkins has not changed."
     News release January 2004.
xi   *insisting that "nothing*: Atkins Nutritionals, Inc. "Frequently asked questions."
     9 August 2004. <http://atkins.com/helpatkins/newfaq/answers/WhyDid-
     DrAtkinsReviseHisNewDietRevolutionDoes.html>.
xi   *can be dangerous*: Shape Up America. "Shape Up America! reveals the truth
     about dieters." News release 29 December 2003.
xi   *largest organization*: Ayoob KT, Duyff RL, and D Quagliani. "Position of the
     American Dietetic Association: Food and nutrition misinformation." *Journal
     of the American Dietetic Association* 102(2002):260–6.
xii *nightmare of a diet*: Frazier A. "Cheers, jeers for no-carb diet: Users like the
     fatty menu, but docs cite dangers." U.S. Senate Select Committee on Nutri-
     tion and Human Needs. "Obesity and fad diets." 12 April 1973:CIS S581-13.
xii *dietitian's nightmare*: Long HL. "Steakhouses craving red-meat Atkins dieters."
     Tampa Tribune 19 October 1999:1.
xii *30 years now*: "Position paper on food and nutrition misinformation on
     selected topics." *Journal of the American Dietetic Association* 66(1975):277–80.

xii   *dietitian talk*: Frazier A. "Cheers, jeers for no-carb diet: Users like the fatty menu, but docs cite dangers." *Chicago Tribune* 18 October 1999.

xii   *My English sheepdog*: Foco Z. "Hype hype hooray: Selling sound nutrition to a country that loves fad diets." *Dietician's Edge* November–December 2001:42–6.

xii   *National Academy of Sciences*: Institute of Medicine. *Weighing the Options: Criteria for Evaluating Weight-Management Programs*. The National Academies Press, 1995.

xii   *American Cancer Society*: American Cancer Society. "Weighing in on low-carb diets." 2004.
<http://www.cancer.org/docroot/SPC/content/SPC_1_A_Low_Carb_Diet_to_ Prevent_Cancer.asp>.

xii   *American Heart Association*: St Jeor ST, et al. "Dietary protein and weight reduction: A statement for healthcare professionals from the Nutrition Committee of the Council on Nutrition, Physical Activity, and Metabolism of the American Heart Association." *Circulation* 104(2001):1869–74.

xii   *Cleveland Clinic*: The Cleveland Clinic. "Weight loss: High protein, low-carbohydrate diets." August 2003. <http://my.webmd.com/content/article/46/2731_1666>.

xii   *Johns Hopkins*: *Johns Hopkins University White Paper: Diabetes 2004*. Simeon, 2004.

xii   *American Kidney Fund*: American Kidney Fund. "AKF warns about impact of high-protein diets on kidney health." News release 25 April 2002.

xii   *American College of Sports Medicine*: Jakicic JM, et al. "American College of Sports Medicine position stand: Appropriate intervention strategies for weight loss and prevention of weight regain for adults." *Medicine and Science in Sports and Exercise* 33(2001):2145–56.

xii   *National Institutes of Health*: National Institute of Diabetes and Digestive and Kidney Diseases. *Choosing a Safe and Successful Weight-Loss Program*. NIH Publ. No 94-3700. National Institutes of Health, Rockville, MD. 1993.

xii   *not seem to be a single*: St Jeor ST, et al. "Dietary protein and weight reduction: A statement for healthcare professionals from the Nutrition Committee of the Council on Nutrition, Physical Activity, and Metabolism of the American Heart Association." *Circulation* 104(2001):1869–74.

xii   *runs counter*: Kappagoda CT, Hyson DA, and EA Amsterdam. "Low-carbohydrate-high-protein diets: Is there a place for them in clinical cardiology?" *Journal of the American College of Cardiology* 43(2004):725–30.

xii   *multi-billion-dollar*: Kahn J. "Wall Street readies for an Atkins feast." *Fortune* 17 May 2004:36.

xii   *official critique*: American Medical Association. "A critique of low-carbohydrate ketogenic weight reduction regimens: A review of Dr. Atkins' Diet Revolution." *Journal of the American Medical Association* 224(1974):1415.
<http://www.AtkinsExposed.org/atkins/75/American_Medical_Association.htm>.

xii   *founder of the Harvard*: Stare FJ and JC Witschi. "Diet books: Facts, fads, and frauds," *Medical Opinion* 1(1972):13–18.
<http://www.AtkinsExposed.org/atkins/96/Fredrick_J._Stare,_Ph.D..htm>.

xii   *current chair*: Blackburn GL, Phillips JCC, and S Morreale. "Physicians' guide to popular low-carbohydrate weight-loss diets," *Cleveland Clinic Journal of Medicine* 68(2001):751.

<http://www.AtkinsExposed.org/atkins/98/George_L._Blackburn,_M.D.,_ Ph.D..htm>.

xiii *dozens of full-text*: "Expert opinions on Atkins."
<http://www.AtkinsExposed.org/atkins/22/Opinions.htm>.

xiii *antique food fad*: Cheuvront SN. "The Zone Diet phenomenon: A closer look at the science behind the claims." *Journal of the American College of Nutrition* 22(2003):9–17.

xiii *factually flawed*: Kennedy ET, et al. "Popular diets: Correlation to health, nutrition, and obesity." *Journal of the American Dietetic Association* 1010(2001):411–20.

xiv *nutritional misinformation*: Cheuvront SN. "The Zone Diet phenomenon: A closer look at the science behind the claims." *Journal of the American College of Nutrition* 22(2003):9–17.

Chapter 1

1 *diet is to be avoided*: Hamilton EMN and EN Whitney. *Nutrition: Concepts and Controversies*. Second Edition. West Publishing Company, 1982:188.

1 Letter on Corpulence: Brody JE. "High-fat diet: Count calories and think twice." *The New York Times* 10 September 2002:F6.

1 *fad melted away*: Deutsch, RM. *The New Nuts Among the Berries*. Bull Publishing Company, 1977:219.

1 *fresh fat meat*: Donaldson BF. *Strong Medicine*. Doubleday, 1960.

2 *worthless scheme*: Fraser L. *Losing It*. Penguin Books, 1997.

2 *Stillman himself died*: Ibid.

2 *ultimate*: Atkins RC. *Dr. Atkins' New Diet Revolution*. Avon Books, 1999.

2 *foolproof*: Agatson A. *The South Beach Diet*. Rodale, 2003.

2 *WORKS 100%*. Atkins RC. *Dr. Atkins' Diet Revolution*. David McKay Company, Inc., 1972:28.

2 *bananas were "poison"*: Ibid:140.

2 *resort entertainer*: Dalton R. "Food fight." *Australian Magazine* 10 April 2004.

2 Tonight Show: Ibid.

2 Merv Griffin Show: Deutsch, RM. *The New Nuts Among the Berries*. Bull Publishing Company, 1977:233.

2 *fastest selling book*: "When a best seller on dieting runs into medical critics." *Modern Medicine* 28 May 1973:132,134.

2 *federal law*: Atkins RC. *Dr. Atkins' Diet Revolution*. David McKay Company, Inc., 1972:295.

3 *Martin Luther King*: Ibid:296.

3 *book was reissued*: Atkins RC. *Dr. Atkins' New Diet Revolution*. Avon Books, 1992.

3 *best-selling fad-diet*: Lenzer, J. "Robert Coleman Atkins: Cardiologist and author of the bestselling diet book in history." *British Medical Journal* 326(2003):1090.

3 *fashion-cult status*: Barrett PH and GF Watts. "Kinetic studies of lipoprotein metabolism in the metabolic syndrome including effects of nutritional interventions." *Nutrition, Metabolism and Cardiovascular Disease* 14(2004):61–8.

3 *Diet Fad of the 21st Century*: Stein K. "High-protein, low-carbohydrate diets: Do they work?" *Journal of the American Dietetic Association* 100(2000):760–1.

3   New York Times Magazine *article*: Taubes G. "What if it's all been a big fat lie?" *The New York Times Magazine* 7 July 2002:22.

3   *billions of media hits*: Topkis M. "The lowdown on low carb: We put Atkins-friendly breads, sweets, and pastas to the test. Which are worth the price?" *Money* 1 December 2003.

3   *$100 million*: Fumento M. "The dangerous legacy of Dr. Atkins." Scripps Howard News Service 24 April 2003. <http://www.fumento.com/fat/atkins.html>.

3   *Atkins advocate*: Squires S. "Experts declare story low on saturated facts." *Washington Post* 27 August 2002: HE01.

3   *$700,000 advance*: Liebman B. "The truth about the Atkins Diet." *Nutrition Action Healthletter* 29(2002):1, 3–7.

3   *simply ignored*: Squires S. "Experts declare story low on saturated facts." *Washington Post* 27 August 2002: HE01.

3   *he ignores them*: Liebman B. "The truth about the Atkins Diet." *Nutrition Action Healthletter* 29(2002):1, 3–7.

4   *It's preposterous*: Ibid.

4   *It was irresponsible*: Ibid.

4   *Taubes sold out*: Fumento M. "Big fat fake: The Atkins Diet controversy and the sorry state of science journalism." *Reason* March 2003.

4   *I was horrified*: Liebman B. "The truth about the Atkins Diet" *Nutrition Action Healthletter* 29(2002):1, 3–7.

4   *during the last 5 years*: Freedman MR, King J, and E Kennedy. "Popular diets: A scientific review." *Obesity Research* 9(2001):1S–40S.

4   *first million copies*: Dorschner J. "New diet book is making a splash: 'South Beach Diet' sells big; cookbook is next." *Detroit Free Press* 11 August 2003.

4   *million dollars a week*: Tanasychuk J. "You've heard of the wildly popular South Beach Diet, but probably not of its creator. A successful cardiologist and an even more successful author, Dr. Arthur Agatston is the . . . man behind the diet." *Sun-Sentinel* (Fort Lauderdale) 11 April 2004:1D.

4   *minus the actual evidence*: "Weighing in on the South Beach Diet." *Tufts University Health and Nutrition Letter* 22(2004):1,8.

5   *own internal inconsistencies*: Ibid.

5   *20 minutes a day*: "Sizing up South Beach." *Harvard Health Letter* November 2003:5.

5   *counting out 15 almonds*: Agatson A. *The South Beach Diet*. Rodale, 2003.

5   *nutrition inaccuracies*: "Weighing in on the South Beach Diet." *Tufts University Health and Nutrition Letter* 22(2004):1,8.

5   *2 grams*: USDA Agriculture Research Service. Nutrient Data Laboratory. National Nutrient Database for Standard Reference. Release 17.

5   *over a third*: Agatson A. *The South Beach Diet*. Rodale, 2003.

5   *nearly as comfortable*: Ibid.

5   *nutrition gaffes*: "Weighing in on the South Beach Diet." *Tufts University Health and Nutrition Letter* 22(2004):1,8.

5   *significantly less saturated fat*: Atkins Health and Medical Information Services . "Atkins challenges copycat diet claims; Atkins experts: 'Show us the science'; Cautions against turning America's health crisis into a fashion war." *PR Newswire* 21 May 2004.

5   *was overweight*: "The Atkins empire strikes back ." *Scripps Howard News Service* 19 February 2004. <http://www.fumento.com/fat/empire.html>.

5   *needs to take medication*: Witchel A. "Doctor wants 'South Beach' to mean hearts, not bikinis." *The New York Times* 14 April 2004:F1.

6   *unbalanced, unsound and unsafe*: "Dr. Atkins' Diet Revolution." *Medical Letter on Drugs and Therapeutics* 15(1973):41.

6   *ridiculously unbalanced and unsound*: "Dietmania." *Medical Times* 107(1979):31.

6   *not been established*: "The Atkins Diet." *Medical Letter on Drugs and Therapeutics* 42(2000):52.

6   *factually flawed*: Kennedy ET, et al. "Popular diets: Correlation to health, nutrition, and obesity." *Journal of the American Dietetic Association* 1010(2001):411–20.

6   *at best half-truths*: Hirschel B . "La révolution diététique du Dr Atkins: Une critique." *Schweizerische medizinische Wochenschrift* 107(1977):1017–25.

6   *scientific literature is in opposition*: Cheuvront SN. "The Zone Diet phenomenon: A closer look at the science behind the claims." *Journal of the American College of Nutrition* 22(2003):9–17.

6   *sprinkling of fallacies*: Dargaville RM. "Food—fads and fallacies." *Australian Family Physician* 6(1977):155–9.

6   *condemning this diet*: "Food faddism." *Nutrition Reviews* 32(1974):53–6

6   *all anecdotal and misleading*. University of California at Berkeley. "Eat fat, get thin?" *Wellness Letter* April 2000.

6   *antique food fad*: Cheuvront SN. "The Zone Diet phenomenon: A closer look at the science behind the claims." *Journal of the American College of Nutrition* 22(2003):9–17.

Chapter 2

7   *Goldman Sachs and Company*: Parthenon Capital. "Parthenon Capital acquires Atkins Nutritionals, Inc." News release 29 October 2003.

7   *talk about its profits*: "Lo-carb, hi finance." *Stanford Business* August 2004.

7   *over two billion dollars*: Kahn J. "Wall Street readies for an Atkins feast." *Fortune* 17 May 2004:36.

7   *Arkansas hog*: Dowdell RW. "Low carb, high profit." *Family Practice News* 34(2004):23.

7   *Hormone That Makes You Fat*: Atkins RC. *Dr. Atkins' New Diet Revolution*. Avon Books, 1999.

7   *monster hormone*: Eades, MR, and MD Eades. *Protein Power*. Bantam, 1997.

8   *single most significant determinant*: Sears B. *Enter the Zone*. Regan Books, 1995.

8   *induce substantial insulin secretion*. SH Holt, Miller JC, and P Petocz. "An insulin index of foods: The insulin demand generated by 1000-kJ portions of common foods." *American Journal of Clinical Nutrition* 50(1997):1264–76.

8   *quarter pound of straight sugar*: Nuttall FQ, et al. "Effect of protein ingestion on the glucose and insulin response to a standardized oral glucose load." *Diabetes Care* 7(1984):465–70.

8   *2 cups of cooked pasta*: SH Holt, Miller JC, and P Petocz. "An insulin index of

foods: the insulin demand generated by 1000-kJ portions of common foods."
American Journal of Clinical Nutrition 50(1997):1264–76.

8   *most insulin secretion*: Ibid.

8   *selectively recite the literature*: Atkins RC, Ornish D and T Wadden. "Low-carb,
low-fat diet gurus face off." Interview by Joan Stephenson. *Journal of the
American Medical Association* 289(2003):1767–8,1773.

8   *only one to significantly lower*: Dansinger ML, et al. "One year effectiveness of
the Atkins, Ornish, Weight Watchers, and Zone Diets in decreasing body
weight and heart disease risk." Presented at the American Heart Association
Scientific Sessions November 12, 2003 in Orlando, Florida.

9   *consistent pattern of higher fasting insulin*: Mayer EJ, et al. "Usual dietary fat
intake and insulin concentrations in healthy women twins." *Diabetes Care*
16(1993):1459–69.

9   *seemed cured of their insulin resistance*: Barnard RJ, et al. "Role of diet and
exercise in the management of hyperinsulinemia and associated atherosclerotic risk factors." *American Journal of Cardiology* 69(1992):440–4.

9   *half the insulin levels*: Toth MJ and ET Poehlman. "Sympathetic nervous system activity and resting metabolic rate in vegetarians." *Metabolism*
43(1994):621–5.

9   *usually doesn't exist*: Sugarman C. "Eat fat, get thin? Dieters on protein-rich
regimens report great success. But some doctors question the safety of these
low-carb plans." *Washington Post* 23 November 1999:Z10.

9   *lose variety and nutrition*: Stein K. "High-protein, low-carbohydrate diets: Do
they work?" *Journal of the American Dietetic Association* 100(2000):760–1.

9   *doesn't make physiological sense*: Liebman, B. "The truth about the Atkins
Diet." *Nutrition Action Healthletter* 29(2002):1, 3–7.

10   *rotten-apple breath*: Langley S. "High protein, low-carb follies: The new fad
diets propagate a lot of myths but the truth is, we already have a key to
weight loss: Exercise." *Health* 19(1996):102.

10   *gallon of water*: Bloom WL and GD Azar. "Similarities of carbohydrate deficiency and fasting: Weight loss, electrolyte excretion, and fatigue." *Archives of
Internal Medicine* 112(1963):333–37.

10   *nauseated or worse*: Blackburn GL, Phillips JC, and S Morreale. "Physician's
guide to popular low-carbohydrate weight-loss diets." *Cleveland Clinic Journal
of Medicine* 68(2001):761, 765–6, 768–9, 773–4.

10   *cash cows*: Bray GA. "Low-carbohydrate diets and realities of weight loss."
Journal of the American Medical Association 289(2003):1853–1855.

11   *$33-billion diet gimmick*: Callaway W. *The Callaway Diet*. Bantam, 1990.

11   *eating fewer calories*: Yudkin J and M Carey. "The treatment of obesity by the
'high-fat' diet: The inevitability of calories." *The Lancet* 2(1960):939–41.

11   *consume fewer calories*: Freedman MR, King J, Kennedy E. "Popular diets: A
scientific review." *Obesity Research* 9(2001):1S–40S.

11   *No magic ingredients*: Roberts DC. "Quick weight loss: Sorting fad from fact."
Medical Journal of Australia 175(2001):637–40.

11   *subnormal intellects*: Atkins RC. *Dr. Atkins' New Diet Revolution*. Avon Books,
1999.

11   *more fat by watching TV*: Sears, B. *Enter the Zone*. Regan Books, 1995.

11   *Goodness, what channel*: Fumento, M. "Fad diet failures." Scripps Howard News Service 13 November 2003. <http://www.fumento.com/fat/study.html>.

11   *5,500 calories a day*: Atkins RC. *Dr. Atkins' Diet Revolution*. David McKay Company, Inc., 1972:93.

11   *bizarre concepts of nutrition*: "A critique of low-carbohydrate ketogenic weight reduction regimens. A review of Dr. Atkins' diet revolution." *Journal of the American Medical Association* 224(1973):1415–1419.

12   *"sneak" calories out*: Atkins RC. *Dr. Atkins' Diet Revolution*. David McKay Company, Inc., 1972:133.

12   *armchair and lose weight*: "The Atkins Diet." *Horizon* (BBC Two) 22 January 2004.

12   *mysterious and magical*: Smith BB. "Doctor sheds two chins—by eliminating carbohydrates." *Houston Chronicle* 9 March 1973.

12   *We found no difference*: Rombeck, T. "KU research has beef with Atkins diet: Professor disputes low-carb regimen's claim." *Journal-World* (Lawrence, KS) 27 January 2004.

12   *No scientific evidence exists*: "A critique of low-carbohydrate ketogenic weight reduction regimens. A review of Dr. Atkins' diet revolution." *Journal of the American Medical Association* 224(1973):1415–1419.

12   *in no way correlated*: Bravata DM, et al. "Efficacy and safety of low-carbohydrate diets: A systematic review." *Journal of the American Medical Association* 289(2003):1837–50.

12   *nothing matters more*: Vigilante KC and MM Flynn. "From Atkins to Zone: The truth about high-fat, high-protein diets for weight loss." *Medicine and Health* 83(2000):337–8.

13   *This whole ketosis thing*: "Dr. Robert C. Atkins: Refighting the battle of the bulge." *The New York Times* 27 November 1996:C1.

13   *listed over 300*: Atkins RC. *Dr. Atkins' New Diet Revolution* Third edition. M. Evans and Company, Inc. 2002.

13   *used ill-defined diets*: Freedman MR, King J, and E Kennedy. "Popular diets: A scientific review." *Obesity Research* 9(2001):1S–40S.

13   *seriously questionable validity*: Grande F. "Energy balance and body composition changes: A critical study of three recent publications." *Annals of Internal Medicine* 68(1968):467–80.

13   *findings of the rest*: Evans E, Stock AL and J Yudkin. "The absence of undesirable changes during consumption of the low carbohydrate diet." *Nutrition and Metabolism* 17(1974):360–7; Yudkin J and M Carey. "The treatment of obesity by the 'high-fat' diet: The inevitability of calories." *The Lancet* 2(1960):939–41; GW Reed and JO Hill. "Measuring the thermic effect of food." *American Journal of Clinical Nutrition* 63(1996):174–9; Golay A, et al. "Weight-loss with low or high carbohydrate diet?" *International Journal of Obesity and Related Metabolic Disorders* 20(1996):1067–72; Alford BB, Blankenship AC, and RD Hagen. "The effects of variations in carbohydrate, protein, and fat content of the diet upon weight loss, blood values, and nutrient intake of adult obese women." *Journal of the American Dietetic Association* 90(1990):534–40; Rickman F, et al. "Changes in serum cholesterol during the Stillman diet." *Journal of the American Medical Association* 228(1974):54–8; Larosa JC, et al. "Effects of high-protein, low-carbohydrate dieting on plasma lipoproteins and body weight. *Journal of the American Dietetic Association*

77(1980):264–70; Fletcher RF, McCririck MY, and AC Crooke. "Reducing diets. Weight loss of obese patients on diets of different composition." *British Journal of Nutrition* 15(1961):53–8; Lewis SB, et al. "Effect of diet composition on metabolic adaptations to hypocaloric nutrition: comparison of high carbohydrate and high fat isocaloric diets." *American Journal of Clinical Nutrition* 30(1977):160–70; Kasper H, Thiel H, and Ehl M. "Response of body weight to a low carbohydrate, high fat diet in normal and obese subjects." *American Journal of Clinical Nutrition* 26(1973):197–204; Bortz WM, Howat P, and WL Holmes. "Fat, carbohydrate, salt, and weight loss. Further studies." *American Journal of Clinical Nutrition* 21(1968):1291–1301; Krehl WA, et al. "Some metabolic changes induced by low carbohydrate diets." *American Journal of Clinical Nutrition* 20(1967):139–148; Young CM, et al. "Effect of body composition and other parameters in obese young men of carbohydrate level of reduction diet." *American Journal of Clinical Nutrition* 24(1971):290–6; Worthington BS and LE Taylor. "Balanced low-calorie vs. high-protein-low-carbohydrate reducing diets. I. Weight loss, nutrient intake, and subjective evaluation." *Journal of the American Dietetic Association* 64(1974):47–51; *International Journal of Obesity and Related Metabolic Disorders* 3(1979):210; Rabast U, Kasper H, and J Schönborn. "Comparative studies in obese subjects fed carbohydrate-restricted and high carbohydrate 1,000-calorie formula diets." *Nutrition and Metabolism* 22(1978):269–77; Baron JA, et al. "A randomized controlled trial of low carbohydrate and low fat/high fiber diets for weight loss." *American Journal of Public Health* 76(1986):1293–1547; Werner SC. "Comparison between weight reduction on a high-calorie, high-fat diet and on an isocaloric regimen high in carbohydrate." *New England Journal of Medicine* 252(1955):661–5.

13   *erroneous data*: Grande F. "Energy balance and body composition changes: A critical study of three recent publications." *Annals of Internal Medicine* 68(1968):467–80.

13   *half of their energy*: USDA Economic Research Service. "U.S. agriculture—linking consumers and producers." <http://www.usda.gov/news/pubs/factbook/001a.pdf>.

14   *does it matter which two*: Fumento M. "Big fat fake: The Atkins Diet controversy and the sorry state of science journalism." *Reason* March 2003.

14   *never gets out*: Dalton R. "Food fight." *Australian Magazine* 10 April 2004.

14   *hamburger fondue*: Atkins RC. *Dr. Atkins' Diet Revolution*. David McKay Company, Inc., 1972:200.

14   *Swiss Snack*: Atkins RC. *Dr. Atkins' New Diet Revolution*. Avon Books, 1992.

14   *"secret manna"*: Hodgman J. "Spice up the Atkins Diet." *Men's Journal* September 2003:33.

14   *matzo ball soup*: Atkins RC. *Dr. Atkins' Diet Revolution*. David McKay Company, Inc., 1972:144.

14   *we got fatter*: Taubes G. "What if it's all been a big fat lie?" *The New York Times Magazine* 7 July 2002:22.

14   *carbs are to blame*: Liebman, B. "The truth about the Atkins Diet." *Nutrition Action Healthletter* 29(2002):1, 3–7.

15   *fraction of our obesity rates*: Khor GL. "Nutrition and cardiovascular disease: an Asia Pacific perspective." *Asia Pacific Journal of Clinical Nutrition* 6(1997):122–42.

15   *closer to 2,000*: Centers for Disease Control and Prevention (CDC). "Trends in intake of energy and macronutrients—United States, 1971–2000."*Morbidity and Mortality Weekly Report* 53(2004):80–2.

15   *guaranteed we'd gain weight*: USDA Economic Research Service. *The Economics of Obesity.* E-FAN-04-004, 2004.

15   *bigger portion sizes*: Abel L. "Somewhere on South Beach." *Journal of the Arkansas Medical Society* 8(2004):255–6.

15   *whopping 350 calories*: Liebman, B. "The truth about the Atkins Diet." *Nutrition Action Healthletter* 29(2002):1, 3–7.

15   *over 3,000 calories*: Center for Science in the Public Interest. "What's at steak?" *Nutrition Action Healthletter* January–February 1997.

15   *wading-pool-sized drink*: Horovitz B. "Portion sizes and fat content 'out of control.'" *USA Today* 20 February 1996:1A.

16   *52 gallons of soft drinks*: American Beverage Association. "Soft drink facts." <http://www.nsda.org/variety/facts.asp>.

16   *primarily consumed in soft drinks*: Bray GA, Nielsen SJ, and BM Popkin. "Consumption of high-fructose corn syrup in beverages may play a role in the epidemic of obesity." *American Journal of Clinical Nutrition* 79(2004):537–543.

16   *exactly parallel*: Gray GA. *An Atlas of Obesity and Weight Control.* Parthenon Publishing, 2003.

16   *enormous amount of very clever*: Abel L. "Somewhere on South Beach." *Journal of the Arkansas Medical Society* 8(2004):255–6.

16   *$2 billion a year*: Lovel J. "Coke, Delta decreased ad spending in 2002." *Atlanta Business Chronicle* 11 April 2003.

16   *10,000 ads*: Barboza D. "Rampant obesity, a debilitating reality for the urban poor." *The New York Times* 26 December 2000:F5

16   *normal response*: Critser G. *Fat Land.* Houghton Mifflin Co., 2003.

16   *how can anyone ignore*: Liebman, B. "The truth about the Atkins Diet." *Nutrition Action Healthletter* 29(2002):1, 3–7.

Chapter 3

17   *the most unutterable nonsense*: Howard P and S Treadwell. "Dr. Atkins says he's sorry." *The New York Weekly* 26 March 1973.

17   *Many of the studies*: Bravata DM, et al. "Efficacy and safety of low-carbohydrate diets: A systematic review." *Journal of the American Medical Association* 289(2003):1837–50.

18   *not a single one*: Dansinger ML, et al. "One year effectiveness of the Atkins, Ornish, Weight Watchers, and Zone diets in decreasing body weight and heart disease risk." Presented at the American Heart Association Scientific Sessions November 12, 2003 in Orlando, Florida; Foster GD, et al. "A randomized trial of a low-carbohydrate diet for obesity." *New England Journal of Medicine* 348(2003):2082–90; Stern L, et al. "The effects of low-carbohydrate versus conventional weight loss diets in severely obese adults: one-year follow-up of a randomized trial." *Annals of Internal Medicine* 140(2004):778–85; Fleming RM. "The effect of high-, moderate-, and low-fat diets on weight loss and cardiovascular disease risk factors." *Preventive Cardiology* 5(2002):110–8.

18   *unimpressive 4% lighter*: Fumento, M. "Fad diet failures." Scripps Howard
      News Service, 13 November 2003.
      <http://www.fumento.com/fat/study.html>.
18   *most weight loss*: Dansinger ML, et al. "One year effectiveness of the Atkins,
      Ornish, Weight Watchers, and Zone diets in decreasing body weight and heart
      disease risk." Presented at the American Heart Association Scientific Sessions
      November 12, 2003 in Orlando, Florida.
18   *had no comment*: Atkins Nutritionals, Inc. "One year effectiveness of the
      Atkins, Ornish, Weight Watchers, and Zone Diets in decreasing body weight
      and heart disease risk." <http://atkins.com/Archive/2003/12/11-
      933145.html>.
18   *formally tested for years*: Ornish D, et al. "Intensive lifestyle changes for rever-
      sal of coronary heart disease." *Journal of the American Medical Association*
      280(1998):2001–7.
18   *without hunger or deprivation*: Freedman MR, King J, and E Kennedy. "Popu-
      lar diets: A scientific review." *Obesity Research* 9(2001):1S–40S.
18   *Another of the yearlong studies*: Ornish D. "Was Dr Atkins right?" *Journal of
      the American Dietetic Association* 104(2004):537–42.
18   *60% more*: Fleming RM. "The effect of high-, moderate-, and low-fat diets on
      weight loss and cardiovascular disease risk factors." *Preventive Cardiology*
      5(2002):110–8.
19   *Less than 2% of vegans*: Spencer EA, et al. "Diet and body mass index in
      38,000 EPIC-Oxford meat-eaters, fish-eaters, vegetarians, and vegans." *Inter-
      national Journal of Obesity* 27(2003):728–34.
19   *third of the American public*: Flegal KM, et al. "Prevalence and trends in obe-
      sity among US adults, 1999–2000." *Journal of the American Medical Associa-
      tion* 288(2002):1723–7.
19   *those eating vegetarian were not*: Kennedy ET, et al. "Popular diets: Correlation
      to health, nutrition, and obesity." *Journal of the American Dietetic Association*
      1010(2001):411–20.
19   *higher resting metabolic rate*: Toth MJ and ET Poehlman. "Sympathetic nerv-
      ous system activity and resting metabolic rate in vegetarians." *Metabolism*
      43(1994):621–5.
19   *earlier studies didn't find*: Berlin P, Melby CL and ET Poelman. "Resting
      energy expenditure in young vegetarian and nonvegetarian women." *Nutri-
      tion Research* 10(1990):39–49.
19   *choosing to eat vegetarian*: Toth MJ and ET Poehlman. "Sympathetic nervous
      system activity and resting metabolic rate in vegetarians." *Metabolism*
      43(1994):621–5.
19   *worse they seemed to do*: Foster GD, et al. "A randomized trial of a low-carbo-
      hydrate diet for obesity." *New England Journal of Medicine*
      348(2003):2082–90; Stern L, et al. "The effects of low-carbohydrate versus
      conventional weight loss diets in severely obese adults: One-year follow-up of
      a randomized trial." *Annals of Internal Medicine* 140(2004):778–85.
19   *award-winning*: Anne M. Fletcher. "Anne M. Fletcher, M.S., R.D., L.D."
      <http://annemfletcher.com/>.
20   *added apples or pears*: Conceicao de Oliveira M, et al. "Weight loss associated

with a daily intake of three apples or three pears among overweight women."
Nutrition 19(2003):253–6.

20   *more fruits and vegetables*: Dreon DM, et al. "A very-low-fat diet is not associated
with improved lipoprotein profiles in men with a predominance of large, low-
density lipoproteins." *American Journal of Clinical Nutrition* 70(1999):412–8.

20   *important strategy for weight loss*: Rolls BJ, Ello-Martin JA, and BC Tohill. "What
can intervention studies tell us about the relationship between fruit and vegetable
consumption and weight management?" *Nutrition Reviews* 62(2004):1–17.

20   *high meat consumption*: Kahn HS, et al. "Stable behaviors associated with
adults' 10-year change in body mass index and likelihood of gain at the
waist." *American Journal of Public Health* 87(1997):747–54.

20   *reverse recent increases*: Kahn HS, et al. "Stable behaviors associated with
adults' 10-year change in body mass index and likelihood of gain at the
waist." *American Journal of Public Health* 87(1997):747–54.

20   *people keep believing*: Sugarman C. "Eat fat, get thin? Dieters on protein-rich
regimens report great success. But some doctors question the safety of these
low-carb plans." *Washington Post* 23 November 1999:Z10.

21   *without the gimmicks*: Levy AS and AW Heaton. "Weight control practices of
U.S. adults trying to lose weight." *Annals of Internal Medicine*
119(1993):661–6.

21   *Americans spend $30 billion*: Institute of Medicine. *Weighing the Options.*
National Academy Press, 1995.

21   *50% less effective*: "Results of new study on low-carb dieters released." *The
Gourmet Retailer* 21 July 2004.

21   *most successful dieters*: Consumers Union. "In the largest survey of its kind,
consumer reports found 83% of the most successful dieters said they lost
weight entirely on their own." News release 17 May 2002.

21   *confirmed to have lost*: Gorman C. "The secrets of their success: Shedding
pounds isn't easy. Keeping them off is harder still. What we can learn from
those who did." *Time Magazine* 7 June 2004:107.

21   *Almost nobody's*: Fumento M. "Big fat fake: The Atkins Diet controversy and
the sorry state of science journalism." *Reason* March 2003.

21   *five times as many carbs*: Klem ML, et al. "A descriptive study of individuals
successful at long-term maintenance of substantial weight loss." *American
Journal of Clinical Nutrition* 99(1997):239–46; Atkins RC. *Dr. Atkins' New
Diet Revolution*. Avon Books, 1999.

22   *believe me, we've tried*: Squires, S. "Experts declare story low on saturated
facts." *Washington Post* 27 August 2002: HE01.

22   *Twenty-six million Americans*: Kadlec D, et al. "The low-carb frenzy." *Time
Magazine* 3 May 2004:46.

22   *plugged in Dr. Atkins' own book*: Atkins RC. *Dr. Atkins' New Diet Revolution*
Third edition. M. Evans and Company, Inc. 2002:364.

22   *Registry demands proof*: Klem ML, et al. "A descriptive study of individuals
successful at long-term maintenance of substantial weight loss." *American
Journal of Clinical Nutrition* 99(1997):239–46.

22   *the BEST feature*: Atkins RC. *Dr. Atkins' Diet Revolution*. David McKay Company, Inc., 1972:289.

22   *tend to fail*: Blackburn GL, Phillips JC, and S Morreale. "Physician's guide to

popular low-carbohydrate weight-loss diets." *Cleveland Clinic Journal of Medicine* 68(2001):761, 765–6, 768–9, 773–4.

23   *current level of ineptitude*: "Robert Coleman Atkins." *British Medical Journal* 326(2003):1090.

23   *money-making proposition*: Dentzer S. "The diet debate." *NewsHour with Jim Lehrer* (PBS) 2 March 2000.

23   *self-aggrandizing*: "When a best seller on dieting runs into medical critics." *Modern Medicine* 28 May 1973:132,134.

23   *revoke his medical license*: "Robert C. Atkins, diet guru and author, dies." *Washington Post* 18 April 2003:B06.

23   *questionable and unproven*: Blackburn GL, Phillips JC, and S Morreale. "Physician's guide to popular low-carbohydrate weight-loss diets." *Cleveland Clinic Journal of Medicine* 68(2001):761, 765–6, 768–9, 773–4.

Chapter 4

24   *55,000 pregnancies*: U.S. Senate Select Committee on Nutrition and Human Needs. "Obesity and fad diets." 12 April 1973:CIS S581-13.

24   *born mentally retarded*: Solomon N. "Improper dieting—a health hazard." *Maryland State Medical Journal* 23(1974):70–3.

24   *considerable concern*: Rudolf MC and RS Sherwin. "Maternal ketosis and its effects on the fetus." *Clinics in Endocrinology and Metabolism* 12(1983):413–28.

24   *all my pregnant patients*: Atkins RC. *Dr. Atkins' Diet Revolution*. David McKay Company, Inc., 1972:288.

24   *I now understand*: Howard P and S Treadwell. "Dr. Atkins says he's sorry." *The New York Weekly* 26 March 1973.

25   *I will stand*: U.S. Senate Select Committee on Nutrition and Human Needs. "Obesity and fad diets." 12 April 1973:CIS S581-13.

25   *small-print disclaimer*: Atkins RC. *Dr. Atkins' New Diet Revolution*. Avon Books, 1999.

25   *extraordinarily irresponsible*: Hamilton EMN and EN Whitney. *Nutrition: Concepts and Controversies*. Second Edition. West Publishing Company, 1982.

25   *Russian roulette*: Mercer M. "The Atkins Diet: Is it safe?" *McCall's Monthly Newsletter for Women* April 1973.

25   *potentially dangerous to everyone*: Smith BB. "Doctor sheds two chins—by eliminating carbohydrates." *Houston Chronicle* 9 March 1973.

25   *"brilliant"*: Atkins RC. *Dr. Atkins' Diet Revolution*. David McKay Company, Inc., 1972:23; Atkins RC. *Dr. Atkins' New Diet Revolution*. Perennial Currents, 2002:65; Atkins RC. *Dr. Atkins' New Diet Revolution*. Avon Books, 1992.

25   *would never "recommend"*: U.S. Senate Select Committee on Nutrition and Human Needs. "Obesity and fad diets." 12 April 1973:CIS S581-13.

25   *symptoms of ketosis*: Blackburn GL, Phillips JC, and S Morreale. "Physician's guide to popular low-carbohydrate weight-loss diets." *Cleveland Clinic Journal of Medicine* 68(2001):761, 765–6, 768–9, 773–4.

26   *physical lack of energy*: Bloom WL and GD Azar. "Similarities of carbohydrate deficiency and fasting: Weight loss, electrolyte excretion, and fatigue." *Archives of Internal Medicine* 112(1963):333–37.

26   *despite what Dr. Atkins claims*: Hirschel B. "La révolution diététique du Dr Atkins: Une critique." *Schweizerische medizinische Wochenschrift* 107(1977):1017–25.

26   *smelled strongly of acetone*: Kark RM, Johnson RE, and JS Lewis. "Defects of pemmican as an emergency ration for infantry troops." *War Medicine* 7(1945):345–52.

26   *significant toxicity*: Ballaban-Gil K, et al. "Complications of the ketogenic diet." *Epilepsia* 39(1998):744–8.

26   *September 2004 review*: Astrup A, Meinert Larsen T, and A Harper. "Atkins and other low-carbohydrate diets: Hoax or an effective tool for weight loss?" *The Lancet* 364(2004):897–9.

26   *most prestigious*: Hutchinson M. "How *The Lancet* made medical history." *BBC News* 6 October 2003.

26   *start to malfunction*: "Atkins diet has long-term dangers, researchers warn." *The Independent* (London) 3 September 2004.

26   *study funded by Atkins*: Yancy WS Jr, et al. "A low-carbohydrate, ketogenic diet versus a low-fat diet to treat obesity and hyperlipidemia: A randomized, controlled trial." *Annals of Internal Medicine* 140(2004):769–77.

27   *at least 30–35 grams*: American College of Gastroenterology. "American Gastroenterological Association medical position statement: Impact of dietary fiber on colon cancer occurrence." *Gastroenterology* 118(2000):1233–4.

27   *from foods, not from supplements*: Krauss RM, et al. "AHA Dietary Guidelines: Revision 2000: A statement for healthcare professionals from the Nutrition Committee of the American Heart Association." *Circulation*. 102(2000):2284–99.

27   *2 grams of fiber*: Atkins RC. *Dr. Atkins' New Diet Revolution*. Avon Books, 1999.

27   *less than 7%*: American College of Gastroenterology. "American Gastroenterological Association medical position statement: Impact of dietary fiber on colon cancer occurrence." *Gastroenterology* 118(2000):1233–4.

27   *answer is supplementation*: Atkins RC. *Dr. Atkins' New Diet Revolution*. Perennial Currents, 2002:76.

27   Annals of Internal Medicine *study*: Yancy WS Jr, et al. "A low-carbohydrate, ketogenic diet versus a low-fat diet to treat obesity and hyperlipidemia: A randomized, controlled trial." *Annals of Internal Medicine* 140(2004):769–77.

27   *misleadingly lauded*: Fumento, M. "Diet disinformation." *The Washington Times* 30 May 2004:B03.

27   *outright dangerous*: Berland, T and L Frohman. *Consumer Guide Rating the Diets*. Publications International, Ltd., 1974.

27   *"Worst Diet"*: Healthy Weight Network. "Year 2000 Slim Chance Awards." <http://www.healthyweightnetwork.com/posters.htm#Slim%20Chance%20Awards%20poster>.

28   *known for its gluttony*: Brewer C. *The Death of Kings: A Medical History of the Kings and Queens of England*. Abson Books, 2000.

28   *essentially every single study*: Freedman MR, King J, and E Kennedy. "Popular diets: A scientific review." *Obesity Research* 9(2001):1S–40S.

28   *independent risk factor*: Rich MW. "Uric acid: Is it a risk factor for cardiovascular disease?" *American Journal of Cardiology* 85(2000):1018–21.

28   *21% increase*: Choi HK, et al. "Purine-rich foods, dairy and protein intake, and the risk of gout in men." *New England Journal of Medicine* 350(2004):1093–103.

28   *blamed directly*: Khan S. "Galloping gout is blamed on fad diets." *The Observer* 18 January 2004.

28   *fit for a prince*: Atkins RC. *Dr. Atkins' New Diet Revolution.* Avon Books, 1999.

28   *muscle cramps or worse.* Bilsborough SA and TC Crowe. "Low-carbohydrate diets: What are the potential short- and long-term health implications?" *Asia Pacific Journal of Clinical Nutrition* 12(2002):396–404.

28   *proper prescription*: *Dr. Atkins' New Diet Revolution* Third edition. M. Evans and Company, Inc. 2002:141.

29   *flawed Zone Diet*: Cheuvront SN. "The Zone Diet phenomenon: A closer look at the science behind the claims." *Journal of the American College of Nutrition* 22(2003):9–17.

29   *something wrong with that*: Stein J. "The low-carb diet craze." *Time Magazine* 154(1999).

29   *significant drop in cognitive performance*: Wing RR, Vazquez JA, and CM Ryan. "Cognitive effects of ketogenic weight-reducing diets." *International Journal of Obesity* 19(1995):811–6.

29   *modest neuropsychological impairment*: Wing RR, Vazquez JA, and CM Ryan. "Cognitive effects of ketogenic weight-reducing diets." *International Journal of Obesity* 19(1995):811–6.

29   *irritable and depressed*: Thomson EA. "Carbs are essential for effective dieting and good mood, Wurtman says." *MIT News* 20 February 2004.

29   *measured the serotonin levels*: Moss L. "Atkins diet 'causes mood swings and depression.'" Press Association 1 March 2004.

29   *MIT researchers found*: Thomson EA. "Carbs are essential for effective dieting and good mood, Wurtman says." *MIT News* 20 February 2004.

29   *most at risk*: Halber D. "MIT researchers: High-carb supplement helps with weight loss." *MIT News* 4 November 2002.

30   *emotional zombie*: Thomson EA. "Carbs are essential for effective dieting and good mood, Wurtman says." *MIT News* 20 February 2004.

30   *take a laxative*: Atkins RC. *Dr. Atkins' Diet Revolution.* David McKay Company, Inc., 1972:153.

30   *calcium deficiency*: Ibid:279.

30   *routinely prescribe a drug*: Ibid:131.

30   *even death*: "Allopurinol." *Physicians' Desk Reference.* Thomson Healthcare, 2004.

30   *working at full efficiency*: Atkins RC. *Dr. Atkins' New Diet Revolution.* Avon Books, 1999.

30   *sweet breath*: Atkins RC. *Dr. Atkins' Diet Revolution.* David McKay Company, Inc., 1972:274.

30   *sunshine and sex*: *Dr. Atkins' New Diet Revolution.* Third edition. M. Evans and Company, Inc. 2002:57.

30   *It's certainly not*: "The Atkins Diet." *Horizon* (BBC Two) 22 January 2004.

31   *handout warning*: Moore CL. "The dangers of self-monitored dieting: What are our patients really doing?" *Cleveland Clinic Journal of Medicine* 68(2001):776.

Chapter 5

32   *serious threat to health*: U.S. Senate Select Committee on Nutrition and Human Needs. "Obesity and fad diets." 12 April 1973:CIS S581-13.

32   *American Heart Association*: St Jeor ST, et al. Nutrition Committee of the Council on Nutrition, Physical Activity, and Metabolism of the American Heart Association. "Dietary protein and weight reduction: A statement for healthcare professionals from the Nutrition Committee of the Council on Nutrition, Physical Activity, and Metabolism of the American Heart Association." *Circulation* 104(2001):1869–74.

32   *type 2 diabetes*: Bilsborough SA and TC Crowe. "Low-carbohydrate diets: What are the potential short- and long-term health implications?" *Asia Pacific Journal of Clinical Nutrition* 12(2002):396–404.

32   *2002 review*: Ibid.

33   *review in the* Lancet: Astrup A, Meinert Larsen T, and A Harper. "Atkins and other low-carbohydrate diets: Hoax or an effective tool for weight loss?" *The Lancet* 364(2004):897–9.

33   *started banning*: Houston S. "Atkins Diet is banned." *Daily Record* 25 August 2003.

33   *Medical Research Council*: Henderson M. "Fat's in the fire as Atkins turns heat on critics." *The Times* (London) 27 September 2003:5.

33   *negligent*: "The weighting game—did the Atkins diet kill Rachel Huskey?" *The Sunday Telegraph* (Sydney) 14 September 2003:51.

33   *nonsense and pseudo-science*: Frith M. "The unpalatable truth about the Atkins Diet: It's just fat-headed nonsense, claim scientists." *The Independent* 13 August 2003:3.

33   *massive health risk*: Prigg M. "Atkins diet is massive health risk says expert." *The Evening Standard* (London) 12 August 2003:D15.

33   *Cleveland Clinic Journal of Medicine*: Blackburn GL, Phillips JC, and S Morreale. "Physician's guide to popular low-carbohydrate weight-loss diets." *Cleveland Clinic Journal of Medicine* 68(2001):761, 765–6, 768–9, 773–4.

33   *real danger of malnutrition*: Kappagoda CT, Hyson DA, and EA Amsterdam. "Low-carbohydrate, high-protein diets: is there a place for them in clinical cardiology?" *Journal of the American College of Cardiology* 43(2004):725–30.

33   *almost went blind*: Hoyt CS III and FA Billson. "Low-carbohydrate diet optic neuropathy." *Medical Journal of Australia* 1(1977):65–6; Hoyt CS and FA Billson. "Optic neuropathy in ketogenic diet." *British Journal of Ophthalmology* 63(1979):191–4.

33   *anti-heart disease properties*: Freedman MR, King J, and E Kennedy. "Popular diets: A scientific review." *Obesity Research* 9(2001):1S–40S.

34   *$640 a year*: Atkins Nutritionals, Inc. "Diet-Pak." <http://atkins.com/shop/products/DietPak.html>.

34   *up to $1,000*: Atkins Nutritionals, Inc. "Anti-Oxidant." <http://atkins.com/shop/products/AntiOxidant.html>.

34   *estimated $400*: Hellmich N. "Can only the rich afford to be thin?" *USA Today* 3 May 2004:2D

34   *$1,400*: " Getting thin on a budget." *The Early Show* (CBS) 25 May 2004.

34   *proper Atkins Dieter*: Atkins RC. *Dr. Atkins' New Diet Revolution*. Avon Books, 1999.

34   *no less than 65*: Kappagoda CT, Hyson DA, and EA Amsterdam. "Low-carbo-
      hydrate-high-protein diets: Is there a place for them in clinical cardiology?"
      Journal of the American College of Cardiology 43(2004):725–30.

34   *chapter entitled "Nutritional Supplements"*: Dr. Atkins' New Diet Revolution.
      Third edition. M. Evans and Company, Inc. 2002.

34   *Who needs orange juice*: Atkins RC. *Dr. Atkins' Diet Revolution*. David McKay
      Company, Inc., 1972:106.

34   *Sue Radd*: "The weighting game—did the Atkins Diet kill Rachel Huskey?"
      The Sunday Telegraph (Sydney) 14 September 2003:51.

34   Cleveland Clinic Journal of Medicine: Blackburn GL, Phillips JC, and S Mor-
      reale. "Physician's guide to popular low-carbohydrate weight-loss diets."
      Cleveland Clinic Journal of Medicine 68(2001):761, 765–6, 768–9, 773–4.

34   *prudent to take*: Volek JS and SC Westman. "Very-low-carbohydrate weight-
      loss diets revisited." *Cleveland Clinic Journal of Medicine* 69(2002):855–62.

35   *as much as 300%*: Willett WC, et al. "Relation of meat, fat, and fiber intake to
      the risk of colon cancer in a prospective study among women." *New England
      Journal of Medicine* 323(1990):1664–72; Giovannucci E, et al. "Intake of fat,
      meat, and fiber in relation to risk of colon cancer in men." *Cancer Research*
      54(1994):2390–7.

35   *colon cancer in 10*: Liebman B. "The sure-fire lightening-fast hunger-free easy-
      as-pie just-4-you permanent-weight-loss health-and-happiness diet." *Nutri-
      tion Action Healthletter*. 31(2004):1, 3–8.

35   *75% greater risk*: Cho E, et al. "Premenopausal fat intake and risk of breast
      cancer." *Journal of the National Cancer Institute* 95(2003):1079–85.

35   *1892*, Scientific American: *Scientific American* 9 January 1892.

35   *American Institute for Cancer Research*: American Institute for Cancer
      Research/World Cancer Research Fund. *Food, Nutrition, and the Prevention of
      Cancer: A Global Perspective*. 1997.

35   *World Cancer Research Fund*: Ibid.

35   *National Cancer Institute*: National Cancer Institute. <http://5aday.gov>.

35   *World Health Organization*: World Health Organization. *Report of the Joint
      WHO/FAO Expert Consultation on Diet, Nutrition and the Prevention of
      Chronic Diseases*. 23 April 2003.

35   *American Cancer Society*: American Cancer Society. "Recommendations for
      nutrition and physical activity for cancer prevention." Revised 21 February 2002.

35   *high-risk option*: American Cancer Society. "Weighing in on low-carb diets."
      2004.
      <http://www.cancer.org/docroot/SPC/content/SPC_1_A_Low_Carb_Diet_to_P
      revent_Cancer.asp>.

35   *risk kidney damage*: Brenner BM, Meyer TW, and TH Hostetter. "Dietary pro-
      tein intake and the progressive nature of kidney disease: The role of hemody-
      namically mediated glomerular injury in the pathogenesis of progressive
      glomerular sclerosis in aging, renal ablation, and intrinsic renal disease." *New
      England Journal of Medicine* 307(1982):652–9.

35   *mild kidney malfunction*: Atkins RC. *Dr. Atkins' Diet Revolution*. David McKay
      Company, Inc., 1972:286.

36   *irreversible scarring*: American Kidney Fund. "AKF warns about impact of
      high-protein diets on kidney health." News release 25 April 2002.

36 *never been reported*: Atkins RC. *Dr. Atkins' New Diet Revolution*. Third edition. M. Evans and Company, Inc., 2002:99.

36 *existed years before*: Brenner BM, Meyer TW, and TH Hostetter. "Dietary protein intake and the progressive nature of kidney disease: The role of hemodynamically mediated glomerular injury in the pathogenesis of progressive glomerular sclerosis in aging, renal ablation, and intrinsic renal disease." *New England Journal of Medicine* 307(1982):652–9.

36 *Harvard Nurses' Health Study*: Knight EL, et al. "The impact of protein intake on renal function decline in women with normal renal function or mild renal insufficiency." *Annals of Internal Medicine* 138(2003):460–7.

36 *high in animal protein*: Coresh J, et al. "Prevalence of chronic kidney disease and decreased kidney function in the adult U.S. population: Third National Health and Nutrition Examination Survey." *American Journal of Kidney Diseases* 41(2003):1–12.

36 *"excessive"*: Kappagoda CT, Hyson DA, and EA Amsterdam. "Low-carbohydrate-high-protein diets: Is there a place for them in clinical cardiology?" *Journal of the American College of Cardiology* 43(2004):725–30.

36 *Plant protein does not*: Goldfarb DS and FL Coe. "Prevention of recurrent nephrolithiasis." *American Family Physician* 60(1999):2269–76.

36 *we would all be vegetarians*: Foreman J. "If you have kidney problems, are you better off avoiding meat?" *Boston Globe* 17 August 2004.

36 *may be exacerbated*: Fleming RM. "The effect of high-, moderate-, and low-fat diets on weight loss and cardiovascular disease risk factors." *Preventive Cardiology* 5(2002):110–8.

36 *worsening of kidney function*: Gin H, Rigalleau V, and M Aparicio. "Lipids, protein intake, and diabetic nephropathy." *Diabetes and Metabolism* 26(2000):45–53.

37 *kidney function was impacted*: American Kidney Fund. "AKF warns about impact of high-protein diets on kidney health." News release 25 April 2002.

37 *wouldn't want to risk it*: Levy A. "Atkins diet 'danger to children.'" *Sunday Mail* (Queensland, Australia) 22 February 2004:27.

37 *Cheese is also a leading source*: Ginty F. "Dietary protein and bone health." *Proceedings of the Nutrition Society* 62(2003):867–76.

37 *solidify into kidney stones*: Herzberg GZ, et al. "Urolithiasis associated with the ketogenic diet." *Journal of Pediatrics* 117(1990):743–5.

37 *significantly increased risk*: Feskanich D, et al. "Protein consumption and bone fractures in women." *American Journal of Epidemiology* 143(1996):472–9.

37 *meat consumption to hip fracture*: Sellmeyer DE, et al. "A high ratio of dietary animal to vegetable protein increases the rate of bone loss and the risk of fracture in postmenopausal women." *American Journal of Clinical Nutrition* 73(2001):118–22.

38 *conceivable complication*: Howard P and S Treadwell. "Dr. Atkins says he's sorry." *The New York Weekly* 26 March 1973.

38 *exaggerated acid load*: Reddy ST, et al. "Effect of low-carbohydrate high-protein diets on acid-base balance, stone-forming propensity, and calcium metabolism." *American Journal of Kidney Diseases* 40(2002):265–74.

38 *even if one includes*: Ibid.

38 *66th*: Atkins Nutritionals, Inc. "Osteo #10." <http://atkins.com/shop/prod-ucts/Osteo_10.html>.

38 *"eaters of raw flesh"*: Bentley DMR. Editorial Emendations to *Abram's Plains: A Poem*, by Thomas Cary. <http://www.uwo.ca/english/canadianpoetry/long-poems/abrams/editorial.htm>.

38 *worst rates of osteoporosis*: Reddy ST, et al. "Effect of low-carbohydrate high-protein diets on acid-base balance, stone-forming propensity, and calcium metabolism." *American Journal of Kidney Diseases* 40(2002):265–74.

38 *2,500 mg per day*: Park YK, Yetley EA, and MS Calvo. "Calcium intake levels in the United States: Issues and considerations." In *Calcium throughout Life.* Food and Agriculture Organization of the United Nations, 1997.

38 *Ice Cream*: Mann GV, et al. "The health and nutritional status of Alaskan Eskimos: A survey of the International Committee on Nutrition for National Defense—1958." *American Journal of Clinical Nutrition* 11(1963):31.

39 *unusually rapid bone loss*: Mazess RB and W Mather. "Bone mineral content of North Alaskan Eskimos." *American Journal of Clinical Nutrition* 27(1974):916–26; Powson IG. "Radiographic determination of excessive bone loss in Alaskan Eskimos." *Human Biology* 46(1974):369–80; Harper AB, Laughlin WS, and RB Mazess. "Bone mineral content in St. Lawrence Island Eskimos." *Human Biology* 56(1984):63–77; Mazess RB and WE Mather. "Bone mineral content in Canadian Eskimos." *Human Biology* 47(1975):45–63; Pratt WB and JM Holloway. "Incidence of hip fracture in Alaska Inuit people. *Alaska Medicine* 43(2001):1–4.

39 *highest levels of these contaminants*: Wormworth J. "Toxins and tradition: The impact of food-chain contamination on the Inuit of northern Quebec." *Canadian Medical Association Journal* 152(1995):1237–40.

39 *finally acknowledge*: Atkins RC. *Dr. Atkins' New Diet Revolution*. Perennial Currents, 2002:130.

39 *serious, potentially life-threatening complications*: Ballaban-Gil K, et al. "Complications of the ketogenic diet." *Epilepsia* 39(1998):744–8.

39 *large part of the diet*: Atkins RC. *Dr. Atkins' New Diet Revolution*. Avon Books, 1999.

39 *shot up to 800*: Tolstol E. "The effect of an exclusive meat diet on chemical constituents of the blood." *Journal of Biological Chemistry* 83(1929):753–6.

39 *Reverse heart disease with filet mignon!*: Atkins Health Revelations Special Report, Winter 2001.

40 *increase LDL cholesterol*: Volek JS and SC Westman. "Very-low-carbohydrate weight-loss diets revisited." *Cleveland Clinic Journal of Medicine* 69(2002):855–62.

40 *single most important risk factor*: Expert Panel on Detection, Evaluation, and Treatment of High Blood Cholesterol in Adults. "Executive Summary of the Third Report of the National Cholesterol Education Program (NCEP) Expert Panel on Detection, Evaluation, and Treatment of High Blood Cholesterol in Adults (Adult Treatment Panel III)." *Journal of the American Medical Association* 285(2001):2486–97.

40 *number one killer*: "National Cholesterol Education Program. Second Report of the Expert Panel on Detection, Evaluation, and Treatment of High Blood

Cholesterol in Adults (Adult Treatment Panel II)." *Circulation* 89(1994):1333–445.

40 *without ever publishing*: Atkins V. "The Robert C. Atkins, M.D., issue." *Metabolic Syndrome and Related Disorders* 1(2003):183–4.

40 *don't bother to read*: Atkins RC. *Dr. Atkins' New Diet Revolution.* Third edition. M. Evans and Company, Inc. 2002:xiii.

40 *prevention of cholesterol elevations*: Atkins RC. *Dr. Atkins' New Diet Revolution.* Avon Books, 1999.

40 *in essence repeated*: Atkins Nutritionals, Inc. "How will doing Atkins help to lower my cholesterol?" <http://atkins.com/helpatkins/newfaq/answers/HowWillDoingAtkinsHelp-ToLowerMyCholesterol.html>.

41 *briefcase I lost*: Berland T and the editors of Consumer Guide. *Rating the Diets.* Rand McNally, 1974.

41 *every single controlled study*: Larosa JC, et al. "Effects of high-protein, low-carbohydrate dieting on plasma lipoproteins and body weight." *Journal of the American Dietetic Association* 77(1980):264–70; SB Lewis, et al. "Effect of diet composition on metabolic adaptations to hypocaloric nutrition: Comparison of high carbohydrate and high fat isocaloric diets." *American Journal of Clinical Nutrition* 30(1977):160–70; Evans E, Stock AL, and J Yudkin. "The absence of undesirable changes during consumption of the low carbohydrate diet." *Nutrition and Metabolism* 17(1974):360–7; Freedman MR, King J, and E Kennedy. "Popular diets: A scientific review." *Obesity Research* 9(2001):1S-40S; Sharman MJ, et al. "A ketogenic diet favorably affects serum biomarkers for cardiovascular disease in normal-weight men." *Journal of Nutrition* 132(2002):1879–85; Sondike SB, Copperman N, and MS Jacobson. "Effects of a low-carbohydrate diet on weight loss and cardiovascular risk factor in overweight adolescents." *Journal of Pediatrics* 142(2003):253–8; Samaha FF, et al. "A low-carbohydrate as compared with a low-fat diet in severe obesity." *New England Journal of Medicine* 348(2003):2074–81; Stern L, et al. "The effects of low-carbohydrate versus conventional weight loss diets in severely obese adults: One-year follow-up of a randomized trial." *Annals of Internal Medicine* 140(2004):778–85; Foster GD, et al. "A randomized trial of a low-carbohydrate diet for obesity." *New England Journal of Medicine* 348(2003):2082–90; Brehm BJ, et al. "A randomized trial comparing a very low carbohydrate diet and a calorie-restricted low fat diet on body weight and cardiovascular risk factors in healthy women." *Journal of Clinical Endocrinology and Metabolism* 88(2003):1617–23; Yancy WS Jr, et al. "A low-carbohydrate, ketogenic diet versus a low-fat diet to treat obesity and hyperlipidemia: A randomized, controlled trial." *Annals of Internal Medicine* 140(2004):769–77; Sharman MJ, et al. "Very low-carbohydrate and low-fat diets affect fasting lipids and postprandial lipemia differently in overweight men." *Journal of Nutrition* 134(2004):8805; Volek JS, et al. "An isoenergetic very low carbohydrate diet improves serum HDL cholesterol and triacylglycerol concentrations, the total cholesterol to HDL cholesterol ratio and postprandial glycemic responses compared with a low fat diet in normal weight, normolipidemic women." *Journal of Nutrition* 133(2003):2756–61.

41 *temporarily decreases*: Di Buono M, et al. "Weight loss due to energy restric-

tion suppresses cholesterol biosynthesis in overweight, mildly hypercholesterolemic men." *Journal of Nutrition* 129(1999):1545–8.

41   should *go down*: Dawson-Hughes B and S Harris. "Effects of weight reduction on blood lipids and lipoproteins: A meta-analysis." *American Journal of Clinical Nutrition* 56(1992):320–8.

41   *shoot through the roof*: Kwiterovich PO Jr, et al. "Effect of a high-fat ketogenic diet on plasma levels of lipids, lipoproteins, and apolipoproteins in children." *Journal of the American Medical Association* 290(2003):912–20; Berkowitz VJ. "A view on high-protein, low-carb diets." *Journal of the American Dietetic Association* 100(2000):1300, 1302–3.

41   *Dr. Jim Mann*: Hall, C. "Atkins dieters 'at risk of sharp rise in cholesterol.'" *Daily Telegraph* (London) 4 September 2003:13.

41   *significantly elevated average LDL*: Volek JS, et al. "An isoenergetic very low carbohydrate diet improves serum HDL cholesterol and triacylglycerol concentrations, the total cholesterol to HDL cholesterol ratio and postprandial glycemic responses compared with a low fat diet in normal weight, normolipidemic women." *Journal of Nutrition* 133(2003):2756–61.

42   *less than 100*: "National Cholesterol Education Program. Second Report of the Expert Panel on Detection, Evaluation, and Treatment of High Blood Cholesterol in Adults (Adult Treatment Panel II)." *Circulation* 89(1994):1333–445

42   *positively frightening*: Yancy WS Jr, et al. "A low-carbohydrate, ketogenic diet versus a low-fat diet to treat obesity and hyperlipidemia: A randomized, controlled trial." *Annals of Internal Medicine* 140(2004):769–77.

42   *investigator concludes*: Fleming RM. "The effect of high-, moderate-, and low-fat diets on weight loss and cardiovascular disease risk factors." *Preventive Cardiology* 5(2002):110–8.

42   *high-fat [Atkins] diets*: Ornish D. "Was Dr Atkins right?" *Journal of the American Dietetic Association* 104(2004):537–42.

42   *cut in half*: Ibid.

42   *average American*: Greenlund KJ, et al. "Trends in self-reported multiple cardiovascular disease risk factors among adults in the United States, 1991–1999." *Archives of Internal Medicine* 164(2004):181–8.

42   *almost heart-attack proof*: O'Keefe JH Jr, et al. "Optimal low-density lipoprotein is 50 to 70 mg/dl: Lower is better and physiologically normal." *Journal of the American College of Cardiology* 43(2004):2142–6.

42   *made the data up*: Squires, S. "Experts declare story low on saturated facts." *Washington Post* 27 August 2002: HE01.

43   *went out of control*: Westman EC, et al. "Effect of 6-month adherence to a very low carbohydrate diet program." *American Journal of Medicine* 113(2002):30–6.

43   *heralded as a vindication*: McConnaughey J. "Two studies vindicate the Atkins diet—but does the weight loss last?" Associated Press 21 May 2003.

43   *probably doesn't kill people*: Fumento M. "Hopeless fad: Sorry, the Atkins Diet still doesn't work." *National Review Online* 6 June 2003. <http://www.fumento.com/fat/nroatkins.html>.

43   *expected to raise coronary heart*: Anderson JW, Konz EC, and DJA Jenkins. "Health advantages and disadvantages of weight-reducing diets: A computer analysis and critical review." *Journal of the American College of Nutrition* 19(2000):578–90.

43   *still gets an F*: Fumento M. "Low carbs and lower journalistic standards." Scripps Howard News Service 27 May 2004. <http://www.fumento.com/fat/media.html>.

43   *2003 "vindication" study*: Samaha FF, et al. "A low-carbohydrate as compared with a low-fat diet in severe obesity." *New England Journal of Medicine* 348(2003):2074–81.

43   *dropped dead*: Stern L, et al. "The effects of low-carbohydrate versus conventional weight loss diets in severely obese adults: One-year follow-up of a randomized trial." *Annals of Internal Medicine* 140(2004):778–85.

43   *widespread fad enthusiasm*: Blackburn GL. "Making good decisions about diet: Weight loss is not weight maintenance." *Cleveland Clinic Journal of Medicine* 69(2002):864–5,869.

43   *on a consistent basis*: Trager S. "Government role in combating obesity." Committee on House Government Reform. *Federal Document Clearing House Congressional Testimony* 3 June 2004.

43   *only a minority*: Sharman MJ, et al. "A ketogenic diet favorably affects serum biomarkers for cardiovascular disease in normal-weight men." *Journal of Nutrition.* 132(2002):1879–85; Sondike SB, Copperman N, and MS Jacobson. "Effects of a low-carbohydrate diet on weight loss and cardiovascular risk factor in overweight adolescents." *Journal of Pediatrics* 142(2003):253–8; Samaha FF, et al. "A low-carbohydrate as compared with a low-fat diet in severe obesity." *New England Journal of Medicine* 348(2003):2074–81; Stern L, et al. "The effects of low-carbohydrate versus conventional weight loss diets in severely obese adults: One-year follow-up of a randomized trial." *Annals of Internal Medicine* 140(2004):778–85; Foster GD, et al. "A randomized trial of a low-carbohydrate diet for obesity." *New England Journal of Medicine* 348(2003):2082–90; Brehm BJ, et al. "A randomized trial comparing a very low carbohydrate diet and a calorie-restricted low fat diet on body weight and cardiovascular risk factors in healthy women." *Journal of Clinical Endocrinology and Metabolism* 88(2003):1617–23; Yancy WS Jr, et al. "A low-carbohydrate, ketogenic diet versus a low-fat diet to treat obesity and hyperlipidemia: A randomized, controlled trial." *Annals of Internal Medicine* 140(2004):769–77; Sharman MJ, et al. "Very low-carbohydrate and low-fat diets affect fasting lipids and postprandial lipemia differently in overweight men." *Journal of Nutrition* 134(2004):880–5; Volek JS, et al. "Comparison of a very low-carbohydrate and low-fat diet on fasting lipids, LDL subclasses, insulin resistance, and postprandial lipemic responses in overweight women." *Journal of the American College of Nutrition* 23(2004):177–84; Volek JS, et al. "An isoenergetic very low carbohydrate diet improves serum HDL cholesterol and triacylglycerol concentrations, the total cholesterol to HDL cholesterol ratio and postprandial glycemic responses compared with a low fat diet in normal weight, normolipidemic women." *Journal of Nutrition* 133(2003):2756–61; GW Reed and JO Hill. "Measuring the thermic effect of food." *American Journal of Clinical Nutrition* 63(1996):174–9; Larosa JC, et al. "Effects of high-protein, low-carbohydrate dieting on plasma lipoproteins and body weight." *Journal of the American Dietetic Association* 77(1980):264–70; SB Lewis, et al. "Effect of diet composition on metabolic adaptations to hypocaloric nutrition: Comparison of high carbohydrate and

high fat isocaloric diets." *American Journal of Clinical Nutrition* 30(1977):160–70.

43   *not necessarily healthful*: Brinton EA, Eisenberg S, and JL Breslow."A low-fat diet decreases high density lipoprotein (HDL) cholesterol levels by decreasing HDL apolipoprotein transport rates." *Journal of Clinical Investigation* 85(1990):144–51.

44   *significantly raising HDL*: Braunwald E, ed. *Harrison's Advances in Cardiology.* McGraw Hill, 2002.

44   *borders on malpractice*: Stare, FJ and J Witschi. "Diet books: Facts, fads and frauds." *Medical Opinion* 1(1972):13–8.

44   *opening up clogged arteries*: Ornish D, et al. "Intensive lifestyle changes for reversal of coronary heart disease." *Journal of the American Medical Association* 280(1998):2001–7.

45   *future epidemic*: Fleming RM. "The effect of high-protein diets on coronary blood flow." *Angiology* 51(2000):817–26.

45   *eat a cheeseburger*. Center for Science in the Public Interest. "Don't say cheese: It's not as innocent as it looks." *Nutrition Action Healthletter* January–February 2001:1.

46   *This couldn't be worse*: Lawrence J. "High fat, low carbs, what's the harm?" *CBS Healthwatch* December 1999. <http://www.lowcarb.ca/articlesa/article235.html>.

46   *stopped in time*: Best TH, et al. "Cardiac complications in pediatric patients on the ketogenic diet." *Neurology* 54(2000):2328–30.

46   *Atkins Corporation denies*: Atkins V. "Statement by Veronica Atkins on the illegal distribution of personal medical information regarding her late husband, Dr. Robert C. Atkins." <http://atkins.com/about/recentnews/wsjresponse.html>.

46   *encourages foods*: "Low-carb, high-protein craze." *American Institute for Cancer Research Newsletter* 67(2000):11.

46   *increased risk of cancer*: American Institute for Cancer Research/World Cancer Research Fund. *Food, Nutrition, and the Prevention of Cancer: A Global Perspective.* 1997; Cho E, et al. "Premenopausal fat intake and risk of breast cancer." *Journal of the National Cancer Institute* 95(2003):1079–85.

46   *diabetes, and heart disease*: Report of a Joint WHO/FAO Expert Consultation. *Diet, Nutrition and the Prevention of Chronic Diseases.* WHO Technical Report Series 916, 2003.

46   *For over 40 years*: Connor WE. "Dietary cholesterol and the pathogenesis of atherosclerosis." *Geriatrics* (1961):407–15.

46   *meat consumption itself*: Snowdon DA, Phillips RL, and GE Fraser. "Meat consumption and fatal ischemic heart disease." *Preventive Medicine* 13(1984):490–500.

46   *"overwhelming"*: AH Lichtenstein and LV Horn. "Very low fat diets." *Circulation* 98(1998):935–9.

46   *Meatless Mondays*: Meatless Mondays. "About us." <http://www.meatlessmondays.com/aboutmm.html>.

47   *deeply concerned*: "A critique of low-carbohydrate ketogenic weight reduction regimens. A review of Dr. Atkins' diet revolution." *Journal of the American Medical Association* 224(1973):1415–1419.

47   *Russian roulette*: Mayer J. "Diet revolution: Basically old hat." *Washington Post* 14 April 1973.

47   *20% of calories*: "Make that steak a bit smaller, Atkins advises today's dieters." *The New York Times* 18 January 2004.

47   *nearly every major health organization*: "National Cholesterol Education Program. Second Report of the Expert Panel on Detection, Evaluation, and Treatment of High Blood Cholesterol in Adults (Adult Treatment Panel II)." *Circulation* 89(1994):1333–445.

47   *misconstruing*: *The New York Times* 18 January 2004.

47   *There is no limit*: Atkins RC. *Dr. Atkins' Diet Revolution*. David McKay Company, Inc., 1972:136.

47   *as much as you want*: Ibid.

47   *no limit on the amount*: Atkins RC. *Dr. Atkins' New Diet Revolution*. Avon Books, 1999.

48   *nothing to do with science*: *The New York Times* 18 January 2004.

48   *Absolutely*: Heimowitz C. "The truth about fat." <http://atkins.com/Archive/2004/2/3-915798.html>.

48   *arteries were clean*: Jody Gorran, Plaintiff, v. Atkins Nutritionals, Inc., and Paul D. Wolff, solely in his representative capacity as co-executor of the estate of Robert C. Atkins, M.D., defendants. County Court of Palm Beach County, Florida. 26 May 2004.

48   *may be hazardous*: Ibid.

48   *million-dollar class action suit*: Smith BB. "Doctor sheds two chins—by eliminating carbohydrates." *Houston Chronicle* 9 March 1973.

49   *without regard to the safety*: "'Diet Revolution' author is sued for $7 million on heart attack." *The New York Times* 23 March 1973.

49   *in favor of the plaintiffs*: Herbert, V. *Nutrition Cultism*. George F. Stickley Co., 1980.

49   *For his ego*: Lauer M. "Jody Gorran, suing Atkins estate, and Dr. Stuart Trager, Atkins nutritional medical director, discuss the possible benefits and hazards of the Atkins diet." *Today Show* (NBC) 28 May 2004.

49   *should not kill you*: Gibson C and D Sawyer. "Man sues Atkins group." *Good Morning America* (ABC) 28 May 2004.

49   *"very strictly"*: MSNBC. *Donahue* 13 November 2002.

49   *Frenzied attempts*: Jones D. "Atkins killed our daughter." *Daily Mail* (London) 23 August 2003:8–9

50   *most likely cause*. Stevens A, et al. "Sudden cardiac death of an adolescent during dieting." *Southern Medical Journal* 95(2002):1047–9.

50   *she should have consulted*: Atkins Nutritionals Inc. "Atkins and independent experts concerned over erroneous news coverage of 2001 death of teen girl." *PR Newswire* 11 November 2002."

50   *lots of near misses*: Henry F. "The skinny on the Atkins Diet." *Newhouse News Service* 5 February 2004.

50   *other people dying*: "The weighting game—did the Atkins diet kill Rachel Huskey?" *The Sunday Telegraph* (Sydney, Australia) 14 September 2003:51.

50   *age of 18 months*: "Power Surge Live! Presents Robert C. Atkins, MD." <http://www.power-surge.com/transcripts/atkins.htm>.

50   *really very dangerous*: "Atkins diet in schools low-carb lessons." *Good Morning America* (ABC) 24 September 2004.

51   *killed our little girl*: Jones D. "Atkins killed our daughter." *Daily Mail* (London) 23 August 2003:8–9.

51   *only three appeared*: Using Lexis-Nexis, searching all-English-language news, no date restriction: "Rachel Huskey" and "Atkins Diet" on 17 May 2004.

51   *die doing something as stupid*: Jones D. "Atkins killed our daughter." *Daily Mail* (London) 23 August 2003:8–9.

51   *"invade Latin America"*: "Atkins Nutritionals ready to invade Latin America." *The Billings Gazette* 18 August 2004.

51   *issued a warning*: Quick D. "One man's meat is another's lentil." *Herald Sun* (Melbourne, Australia) 13 April 2004:16.

51   *bad for people*: Kelly J and F Burstin. "Health alert on diet used by millions." *Herald Sun* (Melbourne, Australia) 15 March 2004:1.

51   *government will distribute*: Ibid.

51   *Australia's chief physician*: Pos M. "Health chief warns on diets." *The Mercury* (Australia) March 16, 2004.

52   *bad for your health*: "Tragic girl who slimmed for love." *The Express* 22 September 2003:6.

52   *much more positive response*: Burstin F. "Dieting empire bares its teeth." *Herald Sun* (Melbourne, Australia) 16 March 2004:12.

52   *only be followed*: Dickerson JW and AM Fehily. "Bizarre and unusual diets." *The Practitioner* 222(1979):643–7.

52   *Congress mandated*: Cooksey K, et al. "Getting nutrition education into medical schools: A computer-based approach." *American Journal of Clinical Nutrition* 72(2000):868S–76S.

52   *less than half*: Soliah L. "Nutrition in medical school curricula." *Today's Dietician* February 2004:21–3.

52   *patients won*: Lazarus K, Weinsier R, and JR Boker. "Nutrition knowledge and practices of physicians in a family-practice residency program: The effect of an education program provided by a physician nutrition specialist." *American Journal of Clinical Nutrition* 58(1997):319–25.

52   *need to be monitored*: Riley RE. "Popular weight loss diets. Health and exercise implications." *Clinics in Sports Medicine* 18(1999):691–701.

52   *According to the chair*: Blackburn GL, Phillips JC, and S Morreale. "Physician's guide to popular low-carbohydrate weight-loss diets." *Cleveland Clinic Journal of Medicine* 68(2001):761, 765–6, 768–9, 773–4.

53   *$10,000–$20,000*: Atkins Nutritionals, Inc. "Diet-Pak." <http://atkins.com/shop/products/DietPak.html>; Atkins Nutritionals, Inc. "Anti-Oxidant." <http://atkins.com/shop/products/AntiOxidant.html>; Hellmich N. "Can only the rich afford to be thin?" *USA Today* 3 May 2004:2D; "Getting thin on a budget." *The Early Show* (CBS) 25 May 2004.

Chapter 6

54   Dateline NBC: "The diet war: Low-fat vs. high-protein with Dean Ornish." 16 July 2002. <http://my.webmd.com/content/article/53/60634.htm?lastselect-edguid={5FE84E90-BC77-4056-A91C-9531713CA348}>.

54   *hydrogenated shortening*: Atkins RC. *Dr. Atkins' Diet Revolution*. David McKay Company, Inc., 1972:137.

54 *should alone improve*: Ascherio A, et al. "Trans fatty acids and coronary heart disease." *New England Journal of Medicine* 340(1999):1994–8.

54 *non-negotiable*: Dr. Atkins' New Diet Revolution. Third edition. M. Evans and Company, Inc., 2002:286.

55 *Krispy Kreme's corporate profits*: Thomson R. "Winners and losers in the food industry as Atkins diet gets huge." *The Evening Standard* (London) 28 May 2004:A49.

55 *under lock and key*: Fumento M and JE Manson. *The Fat of the Land: Our Health Crisis and How Overweight Americans Can Help Themselves*. Penguin, 1998.

55 *Atkins-friendly ice cream*: "Ratings and recommendations for diet meals." *Consumer Reports* 69(2004):12.

55 *Snackwells all over again*: Grayson C. "Low-carb products may jeopardize weight loss efforts." *WebMD Medical News* 10 May 2004.

55 *National Dairy Council admits*: National Dairy Council. "Lactose intolerance and minorities: The real story." <http://www.nationaldairycouncil.org/nutrition/lactose/lactoseIntolerance.asp?page=4>.

55 *most people on the planet*: Hertzler SR, Huynh BC, and DA Savaiano. "How much lactose is low lactose?" *Journal of the American Dietetic Association* 96(1996):243–6.

56 *easy born-again Atkins converts*: "Digestive Disease Week and the 96th annual meeting of the American Gastroenterological Association. San Francisco, California, May 19–22, 1996. Abstracts." *Gastroenterology* 110(1996):A1.

56 *eating one's greens*: Atkins RC. Dr. Atkins' New Diet Revolution. Third edition. M. Evans and Company, Inc., 2002:370.

56 *crumbled fried pork rinds instead*: Atkins RC. Dr. Atkins' Diet Revolution. David McKay Company, Inc., 1972:134.

56 *recent study of 11,000*: NPD Group. "The NPD group reports on low-carb's impact on America's diet." 5 April 2004. <http://www.npd.com/press/releases/press_040405.htm>.

56 *Another survey*: Shape Up America. "Shape Up America! reveals the truth about dieters." News release 29 December 2003.

56 *steak was a carbohydrate*: Henry F. "The skinny on the Atkins Diet." Newhouse News Service 5 February 2004.

57 *no and no*: "Is it possible to follow the Atkins Diet healthfully?" *Tufts University Health and Nutrition Letter* 21(2003):1, 4–5.

57 *highly attractive*: Sugarman C. "Eat fat, get thin? Dieters on protein-rich regimens report great success. But some doctors question the safety of these low-carb plans." *Washington Post* 23 November 1999:Z10.

58 *care more about how*: Ibid.

58 *kills prematurely*: Institute of Medicine. *Weighing the Options*. National Academy Press, 1995.

58 *hundreds of thousands*: Rana JS, et al. "Obesity and the risk of death after acute myocardial infarction." *American Heart Journal* 147(2004):841–6; Stevens J, et al. "The effect of age on the association between body-mass index and mortality." *New England Journal of Medicine* 338(1998):1–7; Fontaine KR, et al. "Years of life lost due to obesity." *Journal of the American Medical Association* 289(2003):187–93.

58 Consumer Guide: Berland T and the editors of Consumer Guide. *Rating the Diets*. Rand McNally, 1974.

58   *"bad boy of diets"*: "Is the Atkins diet on to something?" *Harvard Health Letter* 28(2003):1.

58   *fried eggs and bacon*: Long KH. "Steakhouses craving red-meat Atkins dieters." *Tampa Tribune* (Florida) 19 October 1999:1.

58   *is killing them*: Fumento M. "Big fat fake: The Atkins Diet controversy and the sorry state of science journalism." *Reason* March 2003.

58   *stall*: "Developing countries attack U.N. strategy on obesity." *UN Wire*. 10 February 2004. <http://www.unwire.org/UNWire/20040210/449_12957.asp>.

58   *sabotage*: "U.S. opposes WHO's anti-obesity campaign." *UN Wire*. 16 January 2004. <http://www.unwire.org/UNWire/20040116/449_12157.asp>.

58   *similar tactics*: Centre for Science in the Public Interest letter to Mr. Ed Aiston, Director, General International Affairs Directorate. 16 February 2004. <http://cspinet.org/canada/who_glstrat.html>.

59   Harvard Health Letter: "Is the Atkins diet on to something?" *Harvard Health Letter* 28(2003):1.

59   *not a healthy way*: World Health Organization. "World Health Assembly raises global public health to new level." 22 May 2004. <http://www.who.int/media-centre/releases/2004/wha4/en/>.

59   *increasing the consumption*: World Health Organization. "Frequently asked questions about the WHO global strategy on diet, physical activity and health." <http://www.who.int/dietphysicalactivity/faq/en/>.

59   *"overwhelming"*: AH Lichtenstein and LV Horn. "Very low fat diets." *Circulation* 98(1998):935–9.

59   *refined grains*: Jacobs DR, et al. "Fiber from whole grains, but not refined grains, is inversely associated with all-cause mortality in older women: The Iowa Women's Health Study." *Journal of the American College of Nutrition* 19(2000)326S–30S.

59   *Every single long-term*: Hu FB and WC Willett. "Optimal diets for prevention of coronary heart disease." *Journal of the American Medical Association* 288(2002):2569–78.

59   *lower their risk*: Liu S, et al. "Whole-grain consumption and risk of coronary heart disease: results from the Nurses' Health Study." *American Journal of Clinical Nutrition* 70(1999)412–9.

59   *more than half*: Fung TT, et al. "Whole-grain intake and the risk of type 2 diabetes: A prospective study in men." *American Journal of Clinical Nutrition* 76(2002):535–40.

60   *Fruit consumption*: Willett WC and D Trichopoulos. "Nutrition and cancer: A summary of the evidence." *Cancer Causes and Control* 7(1996):178–80.

60   *reduce heart disease mortality*: Key TJ, et al. "Dietary habits and mortality in 11,000 vegetarians and health conscious people: Results of a 17 year follow up." *British Medical Journal* 313(1996):775–9.

60   *literally millions of deaths*: World Health Organization. "Fruit, vegetables and NCD prevention."<http://www.who.int/dietphysicalactivity/publications/facts/fruit/en/>.

60   *more fruits and veggies*: National Cancer Institute. <http://www.9aday.cancer.gov>.

60   *number one rated*. "About the Wellness Letter." *UC Berkeley Wellness Letter*. <http://www.berkeleywellness.com/html/wl/wlAbout.html>.

60   *"Bottom Line"*: University of California at Berkeley. "Eat fat, get thin?" *Wellness Letter* April 2000.

60   *basics of healthy eating*: Berkowitz VJ. "A view on high-protein, low-carb diets." *Journal of the American Dietetic Association* 100(2000):1300, 1302–3.

61   *Okinawan Japanese*: "Aging: Living to 100: What's the secret?" *Harvard Health Letter* January 2002.

61   *Adventist vegetarians*: Fraser GE and DJ Shavlik. "Ten years of life: Is it a matter of choice?" *Archives of Internal Medicine* 161(2001):1645–52.

61   *Atkins blamed*: "Interview with Robert Atkins." *Larry King Live* (CNN) 6 January 2003.

61   *Fewer than 20%*: U.S. Department of Health and Human Services. Office of the Surgeon General. "The Surgeon General's call to action to prevent and decrease overweight and obesity." 2001.

61   *most successful*: Freedman MR, King J, and E Kennedy. "Popular diets: A scientific review." *Obesity Research* 9(2001):1S–40S.

61   *eating nuts*: Sabate J. "Nut consumption and body weight." *American Journal of Clinical Nutrition* 78(2003):647S–50S.

61   *too much food*: Schaefer EJ, et al. "Body weight and low-density lipoprotein cholesterol changes after consumption of a low-fat ad libitum diet." *Journal of the American Medical Association* 274(1995):1450–5; Siggaard R, Raben A, and A Astrup. "Weight loss during 12 week's ad libitum carbohydrate-rich diet in overweight and normal-weight subjects at a Danish work site." *Obesity Research* 4(1996):347–56; Hays NP, et al. "Effects of an ad libitum low-fat, high-carbohydrate diet on body weight, body composition, and fat distribution in older men and women: A randomized controlled trial." *Archives of Internal Medicine* 164(2004):210–7.

62   *absolutely the worst diet*: Lawrence J. "High fat, low carbs, what's the harm?" *CBS Healthwatch* December 1999. <http://www.lowcarb.ca/articlesa/article235.html>.

62   *vegetable sources of protein*: Willett, WC, Skerrett, PJ, and EL Giovannucci. *Eat, Drink, and Be Healthy: The Harvard Medical School Guide to Healthy Eating.* Simon and Schuster, August 2001.

62   *Partnership for Essential Nutrition*: "Public health groups warn about risks associated with low-carb diets." *Cardiovascular Week* 19 July 2004:46.

62   *seems to have peaked*: Arndt M. "Dude, where's my carb? Pizza and bread companies discover that there's life after Atkins." *Business Week* 9 August 2004:57

62   *passing fad*: Tamaki J. "Restaurants gobble up savings as customers cut down on carbs." *Los Angeles Times* 25 July 2004:C1.

62   Fortune *magazine*: Rynecki D. "The 2004 *Fortune* all-star portfolio; Yes, some analysts really are good stock pickers. Here are the ten best ideas from Wall Street's top researchers." *Fortune* 14 June 2004:152.

63   *neither healthy nor effective*: "Survey: Dread of bread diets easing off." *United Press International* 14 July 2004.

63   *now threatening to sue*: Glaister D. "Zeta-Jones 'hysterical' over threats: Court told woman sent 'violent, graphic and disgusting' letter." *The Guardian* (London) 29 July 2004:539.

63   *cattlemen*: Kawar M. "Cattlemen hope Atkins diet boom doesn't go bust." *Omaha World Herald* 28 July 2004:1D.

63   *starts to slip*: Ryan's Restaurant Group. "Ryan's announces second quarter 2004 results." News release 21 July 2004.

63   *poking fun*: Leonhardt N. "Diet another day: A backlash to all the weight-loss obsession has begun to creep into a wide, wry variety of commercials." *Baltimore Sun* 11 July 2004:1D.

63   *wheels started to fall off*: Maich S. "Low-carb bubble: The diet that was supposed to permanently change how we eat is starting to look like a fad after all." *Maclean's* 23 August 2004.

63   *stuck with backlogs*: Kawar M. "Cattlemen hope Atkins diet boom doesn't go bust." *Omaha World Herald* 28 July 2004:1D.

63   *disappointing sales*: Adamy J. "Some food makers trim low-carb plans as trend slows." *Wall Street Journal* 12 July 2004:B1.

63   *over a cliff*: Moukheiber Z. "A low-carb retailing disaster." *Forbes* 26 July 2004.

63   *food-fad effect*: Adamy J. "Some food makers trim low-carb plans as trend slows." *Wall Street Journal* 12 July 2004:B1.

63   *retailers are discounting them.* Schmit J. "Low-carb craze loses insanity, but it's still strong." *USA Today* 3 August 2004:1B.

63   *Layoffs*: Sanger E. "Low-carb craze slows: Lean times for Atkins foods; Company plans layoffs…"*Newsday* (New York) 14 September 2004.

63   *It defied logic*: Davies J. "Losing their appetite: Low-carb craze wanes, but diehards keep niche stores afloat." *San Diego Union Tribune* 27 August 2004.

63   *Wall Street analyst*: Rynecki D. "The 2004 *Fortune* All-star portfolio; Yes, some analysts really are good stock pickers. Here are the ten best ideas from Wall Street's top researchers." *Fortune* 14 June 2004:152.

Addendum

65   *defaming*: Wachtell, Lipton, Rosen and Katz; Booker, LT. "Philip Morris Companies Inc. and Philip Morris Incorporated, Plaintiffs vs. American Broadcasting Companies, Inc., Forrest Sawyer, John Martin, Walt Bogdanich, and John/Jane Doe(s) I-IV, Defendants." 20 Mar 1994. Bates: 2022813330-2022813359.

66   *lead paint was bad*: Rabin R. "Warnings unheeded: A history of child lead poisoning." *American Journal of Public Health* 79(1989):166874.

66   *mere opinion*: Norton, HW. "Letters to the Editors *American Scientist* Vol 47 [That Smoking Causes Lung Cancer Is A Mere Opinion]." Mar 1957 (est.) Bates: HT0004104-HT0004106.

66   *exaggerated*: Ahrensfeld, Thomas F. "Memo for file." 7 Nov 1962 Bates: 1005148463.

66   *undemonstrated*: Lee, Peter N. "Smoking during pregnancy and congenital limb deficiency." 1994 Bates: 500802154-500802157.

67   *American Cancer Society*: The official position statements of all these groups are reprinted online at "Expert opinions on Atkins." <http://www.AtkinsExposed.org/atkins/22/Opinions.htm>.

68   *claim support your diet*: Atkins Nutritionals, Inc. "Research supporting Atkins." <http://atkins.com/science/researchsupportingatkins.html>.

68   *no major governmental*: St Jeor ST, et al. Nutrition Committee of the Council on Nutrition, Physical Activity, and Metabolism of the American Heart Asso-

ciation. "Dietary protein and weight reduction: A statement for healthcare professionals from the Nutrition Committee of the Council on Nutrition, Physical Activity, and Metabolism of the American Heart Association." *Circulation* 104(2001):1869–74.

68   *counter to all the current evidence*: Kappagoda CT, Hyson DA, and EA Amsterdam. "Low-carbohydrate-high-protein diets: Is there a place for them in clinical cardiology?" *Journal of the American College of Cardiology* 43(2004):725–30.

68   *literally hundreds*: Bravata DM, et al. "Efficacy and safety of low-carbohydrate diets: A systematic review." *Journal of the American Medical Association* 289(2003):1837–50.

68   *health benefits of cigarette smoking*: *Journal of Comparative Psychology* 2(1922):371; Grumberg NE, Bowen DJ, and DE Morse. "Effects of nicotine on body weight and food consumption in rats." *Psychopharmacology* 83(1984):93–8; Winders SE and NE Grunberg. "Effects of nicotine on body weight, food consumption and body composition in male rats." *Life Sciences* 46(1990):1523–30; Elrod K, Buccafusco JJ, and WJ Jackson. "Nicotine enhances delayed matching-to-sample performance by primates." *Life Sciences* 43(1988):277–87; Levin ED, et al. "Chronic nicotine and withdrawal effects on radial-arm maze performance in rats." *Behavioral and Neural Biology* 53(1990):269–76; Devor E and KE Isenberg. "Nicotine and Tourette's syndrome." *The Lancet* 8670(1989):1046; Sanberg PR, et al. "Nicotine potentiates the effects of haloperidol in animals and in patients with Tourette syndrome." *Biomedicine and Pharmacotherapy* 43(1989):19–23; Moss DE, et al. "Nicotine and cannabinoids as adjuncts to neuroleptics in the treatment of Tourette syndrome and other motor disorders." *Life Sciences* 44(1989):1521–5; Lashner BA, Hanauer SB, and MD Silverstein. "Testing nicotine gum for ulcerative colitis patients. Experience with single-patient trials." *Digestive Diseases and Sciences* 35(1990):827–32; Sahakian B, et al. "The effects of nicotine on attention, information processing, and short-term memory in patients with dementia of the Alzheimer type." *British Journal of Psychiatry* 154(1989):797–800; Barclay L and S Kheyfets. "Tobacco use in Alzheimer's disease." *Progress in Clinical and Biological Research* 317(1989):189–94; Gothe B, et al. "Nicotine: A different approach to treatment of obstructive sleep apnea." *Chest* 87(1985):11–17; Warburton DM. "Nicotine issues." *Psychopharmacology* 108(1992):393–6; Pritchard WS, Robinson JH, and TD Guy. "Enhancement of continuous performance task reaction time by smoking in non-deprived smokers." *Psychopharmacology* 108(1992):437–42. West R. "Beneficial effects of nicotine: Fact or fiction?" *Addiction* 88(1993):589–90; West R and S Hack. "Effect of cigarettes on memory search and subjective ratings." *Pharmacology, Biochemistry and Behavior* 38(1991):281–6; Warburton DM. "Nicotine: An addictive substance or a therapeutic agent?" *Progress in Drug Research* 33(1989):9–41; Pomerleau OF, Turk DC, and JB Fertig. "The effects of cigarette smoking on pain and anxiety." *Addictive Behaviors* 9(1984):265–71; Sherwood N, Kerr JS, and I Hindmarch. "Psychomotor performance in smokers following single and repeated doses of nicotine gum." *Psychopharmacology* 108(1992):432–6; Kerr JS, Sherwood N, and I Hindmarch. "Separate and combined effects of the social drugs on psychomotor

performance." *Psychopharmacology* 104(1991):113; Jones GM, et al. "Effects of acute subcutaneous nicotine on attention, information processing and short-term memory in Alzheimer's disease." *Psychopharmacology* 108(1992):485–94; Warburton DM, Rusted JM, and J Fowler. "A comparison of the attentional and consolidation hypotheses for the facilitation of memory by nicotine." *Psychopharmacology* 108(1992):443–7; Spilich GJ, June L, and J Renner. "Cigarette smoking and cognitive performance." *British Journal of Addiction* 87(1992):1313–26; Perkins KA, et al. " 'Paradoxical' effects of smoking on subjective stress versus cardiovascular arousal in males and females." *Pharmacology, Biochemistry and Behavior* 42(1992):301–11; Jarvik ME. "Beneficial effects of nicotine." *British Journal of Addiction* 86(1991):571–5; *Journal of Smoking Related Disorders* 3(1992):43; Dursun SM and S Kutcher. "Smoking, nicotine, and psychiatric disorders: Evidence for therapeutic role, controversies and implications for future research." *Medical Hypotheses* 52(1999):101–9; Dickerson TJ and KD Janda. "Glycation of the amyloid beta-protein by a nicotine metabolite: A fortuitous chemical dynamic between smoking and Alzheimer's disease." *Proceedings of the National Academy of Sciences of the United States of America* 100(2003):8182–7; Cosnes, J, et al. "Gender differences in the response of colitis to smoking." *Clinical Gastroenterology and Hepatology* 2(2004):41–8; Froom P, Melamed S, and J Benbassat. "Smoking cessation and weight gain." *Journal of Family Practice* 46(1998):460–4; Warburton, DM and AC Walters. "Attentional Processing." In Ney, T and A Gale (eds) *Smoking and Human Behavior*. Wiley, 1989; Ross RK, et al. "Risk factors for uterine fibroids: Reduced risk associated with oral contraceptives." *British Medical Journal* 293(1986):359–62; Vellacott ID, Cooke EJA, and CE James. "Nausea and vomiting in early pregnancy." *International Journal of Gynecology* 27(1988):57–62; Andersch B and I Milsom. "An epidemiologic study of young women with dysmenorrhea." *American Journal of Obstetrics and Gynecology* 144(1982):655–60.

68   *showing benefits from thalidomide*: Boughman RP. "Thalidomide for chronic sarcoidosis." *Chest* 122(2002):227–32.; Lehman TJ, Striegel KH, and KB Onel. "Thalidomide therapy for recalcitrant systemic onset juvenile rheumatoid arthritis." *Journal of Pediatrics* 140(2002):125–7; "Lichen planopilaris treated with thalidomide." *Journal of the American Academy of Dermatology* 45(2001):965–6; Rajkumar SV, Fonseca R, and TE Witzig. "Complete resolution of reflex sympathetic dystrophy with thalidomide treatment." *Archives of Internal Medicine* 161(2001):2502–3; Lee L, Lawford R, and HP McNeil. "The efficacy of thalidomide in severe refractory seronegative spondylarthropathy: Comment on the letter by Breban et al." *Arthritis and Rheumatism* 44(2001):2456–8; Bousvaros A and B Mueller. "Thalidomide in gastrointestinal disorders." *Drugs* 61(2001):777–87; Camisa C and JL Popovsky. "Effective treatment of oral erosive lichen planus with thalidomide." *Archives of Dermatology* 136(2000):1442–3; Cohen MH. "Thalidomide in the treatment of high-grade gliomas." *Journal of Clinical Oncology* 18(2000):3453; Andrea AG, et al. "Clinical and immunological benefit of adjuvant therapy with thalidomide in the treatment of tuberculosis disease." *AIDS* 14(2000):1859–61; Peuckmann V, Fisch M, and E Bruera. "Potential novel uses of thalidomide: Focus on palliative care." *Drugs* 60(2000):273–92; Burrows NP. "Diagnosis and manage-

ment of systemic lupus erythematosus. Thalidomide modifies disease." *British Medical Journal* 307(1993):939–40; DeVincenzo JP and SK Burche. "Prolonged thalidomide therapy for human immunodeficiency virus—associated recurrent severe esophageal and oral aphthous ulcers." *Pediatric Infectious Disease Journal* 15(1996):4657; Powell RJ. "New roles for thalidomide." *British Medical Journal* 313(1996):377–8; Dereure O, Basset-Seguin N, and JJ Guilhou. "Erosive lichen planus: Dramatic response to thalidomide." *Archives of Dermatology* 132(1996):1392–3; Marwick C. "Thalidomide back—under strict control." *Journal of the American Medical Association* 278(1997):1135–7; Rousseau L, et al. "Cutaneous sarcoidosis successfully treated with low doses of thalidomide." *Archives of Dermatology* 134(1998):1045–6; Raje N and K Anderson. "Thalidomide—a revival story." *New England Journal of Medicine* 341(1999):1606–9; Kumar S, Witzig TE, and SV Rajkumar. "Thalidomide: Current role in the treatment of non-plasma cell malignancies." *Journal of Clinical Oncology* 22(2004):2477–88; Richardson P, et al. "Thalidomide for patients with relapsed multiple myeloma after high-dose chemotherapy and stem cell transplantation: Results of an open-label multicenter phase 2 study of efficacy, toxicity, and biological activity." *Mayo Clinic Proceedings* 79(2004):875–82; Waage A, et al, and the Nordic Myeloma Study Group. "Early response predicts thalidomide efficiency in patients with advanced multiple myeloma." *British Journal of Haematology* 125(2004):149–55; Bauditz J, et al. "Thalidomide for treatment of severe intestinal bleeding." *Gut* 53(2004):609–12; Caradonna S and H Jacobe. "Thalidomide as a potential treatment for scleromyxedema." *Archives of Dermatology* 140(2004):277–80; Yasui K, et al. "Thalidomide therapy for juvenile-onset entero-Behcet disease." *Journal of Pediatrics* 143(2003):692–4; Thomas DA, et al. "Single agent thalidomide in patients with relapsed or refractory acute myeloid leukaemia." *British Journal of Haematology* 123(2003):436–41; Hernberg M, et al. "Interferon Alfa-2b three times daily and thalidomide in the treatment of metastatic renal cell carcinoma." *Journal of Clinical Oncology* 21(2003):3770–6; Schwartzman RJ, Chevlen E, and K Bengtson. "Thalidomide has activity in treating complex regional pain syndrome." *Archives of Internal Medicine* 163(2003):1487; Loprinzi C and SV Rajkumar. "Why not start with thalidomide?" *Journal of Clinical Oncology* 21(2003):2211–4; Younis TH, et al. "Reversible pulmonary hypertension and thalidomide therapy for multiple myeloma." *British Journal of Haematology* 121(2003):191–2; Kumar S, et al. "Response rate, durability of response, and survival after thalidomide therapy for relapsed multiple myeloma." *Mayo Clinic Proceedings* 78(2003):34–9; Mann DL. "Inflammatory mediators and the failing heart: Past, present, and the foreseeable future." *Circulation Research* 91(2002):988–98; Gullestad L, et al. "Effect of thalidomide in patients with chronic heart failure." *American Heart Journal* 144(2002):847–50; Gupta A, et al. "Phase I study of thalidomide for the treatment of plexiform neurofibroma in neurofibromatosis 1." *Neurology* 60(2003):130–2; Weber D, et al. "Thalidomide alone or with dexamethasone for previously untreated multiple myeloma." *Journal of Clinical Oncology* 21(2003):16–19; Jacobson JM, et al. "Thalidomide for the treatment of esophageal aphthous ulcers in patients with human immunodeficiency virus infection. National Institute of Allergy and Infectious Disease AIDS Clinical Trials Group." *Journal of Infectious Diseases* 180(1999):61–7.

68   *downplaying the risks of asbestos*: The Asbestos Institute. <http://www.asbestos-institute.ca/main.html>.

68   *chemical manufacturer's website*: Environmental Working Group. "Arsenic in pressure treated lumber." <http://www.ewg.org/issues/arsenic/index.php>.

68   *children's playgrounds*: Wood Preservative Science Council. "Scientific Reports." <http://www.woodpreservativescience.org/reports.shtml>.

68   *practice now banned*: U.S. Environmental Protection Agency. "Guidance for uses of chromated copper arsenate." 6 June 2004.

68   *supported by pesticide makers*: Center for Media and Democracy. "American Council on Science and Health." <http://www.prwatch.org/improp/acsh.html>.

68   *downplaying the risks of DDT*: American Council on Science and Health. *Facts Versus Fears*. <http://www.acsh.org/publications/pubID.154/pub_detail.asp>.

69   *more than a hundred*: Baron JA. "Beneficial effects of nicotine and cigarette smoking: The real, the possible, and the spurious." *British Medical Bulletin* 52(1996):58–73.

69   *classic tobacco corporation tactic*: Tobacco Industry Research Committee. "A scientific perspective on the cigarette controversy." <http://tobaccodocu-ments.org/ctr/CTRMN003338-3357.html>.

69   *supporting Atkins*: Atkins Nutritionals, Inc. "Research supporting Atkins." <http://atkins.com/science/researchsupportingatkins.html>.

69   *not published studies*: Boden, et al. "Effects of the Atkins Diet in type 2 diabetes: Metabolic balance studies." 64th session of the American Diabetes Association, #321-OR, 8 June 2004; Dansinger ML, et al. "One year effectiveness of the Atkins, Ornish, Weight Watchers, and Zone diets in decreasing body weight and heart disease risk." Presented at the American Heart Association Scientific Sessions November 12, 2003 in Orlando, Florida; Goldstein T, et al. "Influence of a modified Atkins Diet on weight loss and glucose metabolism in obese type 2 diabetic patients." *Israel Medical Association Journal* 6(2004):314; Greene, et al. "Pilot 12-week feeding weight-loss comparison: low-fat vs. low-carbohydrate (ketogenic) diets." Abstract presented at the North American Association for the Study of Obesity Annual Meeting 2003, *Obesity Research* 11S(2003):95OR; Greene PJ, Devecis J, and WC Willett. "Effects of low-fat vs. ultra-low-carbohydrate weight-loss diets: A 12-week pilot feeding study." Abstract presented at Nutrition Week 2004, 9–12 February 2004, in Las Vegas, Nevada; Nickols-Richardson, SM, Volpe JJ, and MD Coleman. "Premenopausal women following a low-carbohydrate/high-protein diet experience greater weight loss and less hunger compared to a high-carbohydrate/low-fat diet." Abstract presented at FASEB Meeting on Experimental Biology: Translating the Genome, Washington, D.C., 17–21 April 2004; O'Brien KD, Brehm BJ, and RJ Seeley. "Greater reduction in inflammatory markers with a low-carbohydrate diet than with a calorically matched low-fat diet." Presented at American Heart Association's Scientific Sessions 2002, 19 November 2002, Abstract No 117597; Stadler DD, et al. "Impact of 42-Day Atkins Diet and energy-matched low-fat diet on weight and anthropometric indices," *FASEB*

Journal 17(4–5): Abstract of the 12th Annual FASEB Meeting on Experimental Biology: Translating the Genome, San Diego, California, 11–15 April 2003: Abstract No 453.3; Yancy WS, Foy ME, and EC Westman. "A low-carbohydrate, ketogenic diet for type 2 diabetes mellitus." *Journal of General Internal Medicine* 19(2004):110S; Westman EC, et al. "A pilot study of a low-carbohydrate, keto-genic diet for obesity-related polycystic ovary syndrome." *Journal of General Internal Medicine* 19(2004):111S.

69 *unreliable sources*: Relman AS. "News reports of medical meetings: How reliable are abstracts?" *New England Journal of Medicine* 303(1980):277–8.

69 *tobacco industry strategy*: Bero LA and SA Glantz. "Tobacco industry response to a risk assessment of environmental tobacco smoke." *Tobacco Control* 2(1993):103–13.

69 *untrustworthy*: Chalmers I, et al. *Journal of the American Medical Association* 263(1990):1401–5.

69 *Less than half*: Marx WF, et al. "The fate of neuroradiologic abstracts presented at national meetings in 1993: Rate of subsequent publication in peer-reviewed, indexed journals." *American Journal of Neuroradiology* 20(1999):1173–7.

70 *routinely overstate*: Weintraub WH. "Are published manuscripts representative of the surgical meeting abstracts? An objective appraisal." *Journal of Pediatric Surgery* 22(1987):11–3

70 *stimulate dialogue*: Soffer A. "Beware the 200-word abstract!" *Archives of Internal Medicine* 136(1976):1232–3.

70 *media shouldn't even report*: Relman AS. "News reports of medical meetings: How reliable are abstracts?" *New England Journal of Medicine* 303(1980):277–8.

70 *guiding principle*: Rothstein JM. "Caveat emptor and conference abstracts." *Physical Therapy* 70(1990):277.

70 *Avoid using abstracts*: International Committee of Medical Journal Editors. "Uniform requirements for manuscripts submitted to biomedical journals." *Journal of the American Medical Association* 277(1997):927–34.

70 *entirely prohibit authors*: Marx WF, et al. "The fate of neuroradiologic abstracts presented at national meetings in 1993: Rate of subsequent publication in peer-reviewed, indexed journals." *American Journal of Neuroradiology* 20(1999):1173–7.

70 *over a quarter*: Atkins Nutritionals, Inc. "Research supporting Atkins." <http://atkins.com/science/researchsupportingatkins.html>.

70 *26,000 serial titles*: Harvard University. "Countway library collections overview."
<http://www.countway.med.harvard.edu/countway/collections.shtml>.

71 *one in Alabama*: Mary Ann Liebert, Inc. Customer service. Personal communication 13 August 2004.

71 *They don't*: University of Alabama at Birmingham. "Lister Hill Library of the Health Sciences." <http://www.uab.edu/lister/>; University of South Alabama Biomedical Library. <http://southmed.usouthal.edu/library/index.html>.

71 *Index Medicus*: National Library of Medicine. "List of journals indexed in Index Medicus." 2004
<ftp://nlmpubs.nlm.nih.gov/online/journals/ljiweb.pdf>.

71 *12,000 titles*: University of Iowa. "Indexed biomedical journals." <http://www.lib.uiowa.edu/hardin/serials.html>.

71 *member*: The International Network of Cholesterol Skeptics. "List of members." <http://www.thincs.org/members.htm>.

71 *representative*: The International Network of Cholesterol Skeptics. "Medical McCarthyism: Experts dispute opposition to dietary fat." News release 5 September 2002.

71 *still Associate Editor*: Mary Ann Liebert Inc. "Metabolic syndrome and related disorders." <http://www.liebertpub.com/eboard.aspx?pub_id=115>.

71 *featured speaker*: SUNY Downstate Medical Center. "Kingsbrook Conference on Nutritional and Metabolic Aspects of Low-carbohydrate Diets. 18–19 June 2004." <http://www.downstate.edu/kingsbrook/default.html>.

71 *President of your Atkins at Home*: Atkins Health and Medical Information Services. "The Atkins lifestyle takes Broadway thanks to home deliveries." PR Newswire 10 March 2004.

71 *get Atkins meals delivered*: Atkins Nutritionals, Inc. "What is the cost of these programs?" <http://atkinsathome.com/faq.asp>.

71 *your official spokesmen*: Nguyen D. "Meal delivery services attract dieters." Associated Press 20 April 2004.

71 *dedicated its premiere issue*: Atkins Nutritionals, Inc. "*Metabolic Syndrome and Related Disorders* honors Dr. Atkins." <http://atkins.com/Archive/2004/4/16-589668.html>.

71 *organized by Dr. Freedland*: Dandona P. "Editorial." *Metabolic Syndrome and Related Disorders* 1(2003):179.

71 *sad to lose a loved one*: Freedland ES. "A tribute to Robert C. Atkins, M.D." *Metabolic Syndrome and Related Disorders* 1(2003):181–2.

71 *prestigious*: Atkins V. "The Robert C. Atkins, M.D. issue." *Metabolic Syndrome and Related Disorders* 1(2003):183–4.

71 *authoritative*: Mary Ann Liebert, Inc. "Controlled carbohydrate diet approach discussed in special issue of journal in memory of Dr. Robert Atkins." *Business Wire* 29 Jan 2004.

71 *reportedly founded*: Dandona P. "Editorial." *Metabolic Syndrome and Related Disorders* 1(2003):179.

71 *on his behalf*: Atkins V. "The Robert C. Atkins, M.D. issue." *Metabolic Syndrome and Related Disorders* 1(2003):183–4.

72 *published by Atkins-funded researchers*: Greene P, et al. "Pilot 12-week feeding weight-loss comparison: Low-fat vs. low-carbohydrate (ketogenic) diets." Abstract Presented at the North American Association for the Study of Obesity Annual Meeting 2003, *Obesity Research* 11S(2003):95OR; Greene PJ, Devecis J, and WC Willett. "Effects of low-fat vs. ultra-low-carbohydrate weight-loss diets: A 12-week pilot feeding study." Abstract presented at Nutrition Week 2004, 9–12 February 2004, in Las Vegas, Nevada; "Clinical yuse of a carbohydrate-restricted diet to treat the dyslipidemia of the metabolic syndrome." *Metabolic Syndrome and Related Disorders* 1(2003):227–32; Sharman MJ, et al. "Very low-carbohydrate and low-fat diets affect fasting lipids and postprandial lipemia differently in overweight men." *Journal of Nutrition* 134(2004):880–5; Sharman MJ, et al. "A ketogenic diet favorably affects serum biomarkers for cardiovascular disease in normal-weight men." *Journal*

of Nutrition. 132(2002):1879–85; Sharman MJ and JS Volek. "Weight loss leads to reductions in inflammatory biomarkers after a very low-carbohydrate and low-fat diet in overweight men." *Clinical Science* (London), 2004; Sondike SB, Copperman N, and MS Jacobson. "Effects of a low-carbohydrate diet on weight loss and cardiovascular risk factor in overweight adolescents." *Journal of Pediatrics* 142(2003):253–8; Vernon MC, et al. "Clinical experience of a carbohydrate-restricted diet: Effect on diabetes mellitus." *Metabolic Syndrome and Related Disorders* 1(2003):233–7; Volek JS, Gomez AL, and WJ Kraemer. "Fasting lipoprotein and postprandial triacylglycerol responses to a low-carbohydrate diet supplemented with n-3 fatty acids." *Journal of the American College of Nutrition* 19(2000):383–91; Volek JS, et al. "Comparison of a very low-carbohydrate and low-fat diet on fasting lipids, LDL subclasses, insulin resistance, and postprandial lipemic responses in overweight women." *Journal of the American College of Nutrition* 23(2004):177–84; Volek JS, et al. "Body composition and hormonal responses to a carbohydrate-restricted diet." *Metabolism* 51(2002):864–70; Volek JS, et al. "An isoenergetic very low carbohydrate diet improves serum HDL cholesterol and triacylglycerol concentrations, the total cholesterol to HDL cholesterol ratio and postprandial glycemic responses compared with a low fat diet in normal weight, normolipidemic women." *Journal of Nutrition* 133(2003):2756–61; Volek JS and EC Westman. "Very-low-carbohydrate weight-loss diets revisited." *Cleveland Clinic Journal of Medicine* 69(2002):849, 853, 856–8; Westman EC, et al. "A review of low-carbohydrate ketogenic diets." *Current Atherosclerosis Reports* 5(2003):476–83; Westman EC, et al. "Effect of 6-month adherence to a very low carbohydrate diet program." *American Journal of Medicine* 113(2002):30–6; Westman EC, et al. "A pilot study of a low-carbohydrate, ketogenic diet for obesity-related polycystic ovary syndrome." *Journal of General Internal Medicine* 19(2004):111S; Yancy WS Jr, et al. "A low-carbohydrate, ketogenic diet versus a low-fat diet to treat obesity and hyperlipidemia: A randomized, controlled trial." *Annals of Internal Medicine* 140(2004):769–77; Yancy WS Jr, Provenzale D, and EC Westman, "Improvement of gastroesophageal reflux disease after initiation of a low-carbohydrate diet: Five brief case reports," *Alternative Therapies in Health and Medicine* 7(2001):116–9; Kossoff EH, et al. "Efficacy of the Atkins Diet as therapy for intractable epilepsy." *Neurology* 61(2003):1789–91; Yancy YS, et al. "A pilot trial of a low-carbohydrate, ketogenic diet in patients with type 2 diabetes." *Metabolic Syndrome and Related Disorders* 1(2003):239–43.

72   *did not reveal the source*: Bailes JR, et al. "Effect of low-carbohydrate, unlimited calorie diet on the treatment of childhood obesity: A prospective controlled study." *Metabolic Syndrome and Related Disorders* 1(2003):221–5; Boden G, et al. "Effects of the Atkins Diet in type 2 diabetes: Metabolic balance studies." 64th session of the American Diabetes Association, #321-OR, 8 June 2004; Goldstein T, et al. "Influence of a modified Atkins Diet on weight loss and glucose metabolism in obese type 2 diabetic patients." *Israel Medical Association Journal* 6(2004):314; Gutierrez M, et al. "Utility of a short-term 25% carbohydrate diet on improving glycemic control in type 2 diabetes mellitus." *Journal of the American College of Nutrition* 17(1998):595–600; Hays JH, Gorman RT, and KM Shakir. "Results of use of metformin and replace-

ment of starch with saturated fat in diets of patients with type 2 diabetes." *Endocrinology Practice* 8(2002):177–83; O'Brien, KD, Brehm, BJ, and RJ Seeley. "Greater reduction in inflammatory markers with a low-carbohydrate diet than with a calorically matched low-fat diet." Presented at American Heart Association's Scientific Sessions 2002 on November 19, 2002, Abstract ID: 117597.

72   *less than half of major*: Warner TD and JP Gluck. "What do we really know about conflicts of interest in biomedical research?" *Psychopharmacology* 171(2003):36–46.

72   *millions of dollars*: National Philanthropic Trust. "National Philanthropic Trust to administer Atkins Foundation." News release 25 May 2004.

72   *prove Dr. Atkins right*: O'Connell P. "I want to prove Dr. Atkins was right." *BusinessWeek Online* 18 June 2004.

72   *misrepresenting science*: Rampton S and J Stauber. *Trust Us, We're Experts.* Penguin Putnam, 2002.

72   *downplay the risks of asbestos*: Ibid.

72   *Chemical companies fund*: Swaen GM and JM Meijers. "Influence of design characteristics on the outcome of retrospective cohort studies." *British Journal of Industrial Medicine* 45(1988):624–9.

72   *Tobacco corporations fund*: Bero LA and SA Glantz. "Tobacco industry response to a risk assessment of environmental tobacco smoke." *Tobacco Control* 2(1993):103–13.

72   *hand that feeds them*: Hillman AL, et al. "Avoiding bias in the conduct and reporting of cost-effectiveness research sponsored by pharmaceutical companies." *New England Journal of Medicine* 324(1991):1362–5.

72   *hundred times higher*: Barnes DE and LA Bero. "Why review articles on the health effects of passive smoking reach different conclusions." *Journal of the American Medical Association* 279(1998):1566–70.

72   *fund independent scientific research*: Barnes DE and LA Bero. "Industry-funded research and conflict of interest: An analysis of research sponsored by the tobacco industry through the Center for Indoor Air Research." *Journal of Health Politics, Policy and Law* 21(1996):515–42.

72   *internal documents showed*: Bero LA and SA Glantz. "Tobacco industry response to a risk assessment of environmental tobacco smoke." *Tobacco Control* 2(1993):103–13.

73   *"sound science"*: Atkins Nutritionals, Inc. "Atkins Nutritionals, Inc., introduces a healthy alternative to a market flooded with sugar-laden 'nutrition' shakes." News release November 2001.

73   *manipulate the scientific standards*: Ong EK and SA Glantz "Constructing "sound science" and "good epidemiology": Tobacco, lawyers, and public relations firms." *American Journal of Public Health* 91(2001):1749–57.

73   *Atkins Physicians Council*: Atkins Nutritionals, Inc. "Atkins Physicians Council." <http://atkins.com/about/atkins-physicians-council.html>.

73   *Project Whitecoat*: Dyer C. "Tobacco company set up network of sympathetic scientists." *British Medical Journal* 316(1998):1555.

73   *built up networks*: Atkins Foundation. <http://atkinsfoundation.org/grants.asp>; Muggli ME, et al. "The smoke you don't see: Uncovering tobacco industry scientific strategies aimed against

environmental tobacco smoke policies." *American Journal of Public Health* 91(2001):1419–23.

73 *publish non-peer reviewed research*: Drope J and S Chapman. "Tobacco industry efforts at discrediting scientific knowledge of environmental tobacco smoke: A review of internal industry documents." *Journal of Epidemiology and Community Health* 55(2001):588.

73 *deep fragrance of academia*: Chapman S, Carter SM, and M Peters "A deep fragrance of academia: The Australian Tobacco Research Foundation." *Tobacco Control* 12(2003):iii38.

73 *routinely ignored*: Bero LA and SA Glantz. "Tobacco industry response to a risk assessment of environmental tobacco smoke." *Tobacco Control* 2(1993):103–13.

73 *Get real*: Atkins Nutritionals, Inc. "Who says there are no studies?" <http://atkins.com/Archive/2002/11/21-533336.html>.

74 *faced intimidation*: "WHO calls for closer monitoring of commercial interests." *British Medical Journal* 324(2002):8.

74 *deceptive corporate sector*: "Resisting smoke and spin." *The Lancet* 355(2000):1197.

74 *Not a* single *one*: Davidson RA. "Source of funding and outcome of clinical trials." *Journal of General Internal Medicine* 1(1986):155–8.

74 *the same uncanny "coincidence"*: Rochan PA, et al. "A study of manufacturer-supported trials of nonsteroidal anti-inflammatory drugs in the treatment of arthritis." *Archives of Internal Medicine* 154(1994):157–62.

74 *may delay or not publish*: Baird P. "Getting it right: Industry sponsorship and medical research." *Canadian Medical Association Journal* 168(2003):1267–9.

74 *suppress the truth*: Bodenheimer T. "Uneasy alliance—clinical investigators and the pharmaceutical industry." *New England Journal of Medicine* 342(2000):1539–44.

74 *not uncommon*: Chopra SS. "Industry funding of clinical trials: Benefit or bias?" *Journal of the American Medical Association* 290(2003):113–4.

74 *significantly less likely*: Friedberg M, et al. Evaluation of conflict of interest in economic analyses of new drugs used in oncology." *Journal of the American Medical Association* 282(1999):1453–7.

75 *choose inappropriate controls*: Warner TD and JP Gluck. "What do we really know about conflicts of interest in biomedical research?" *Psychopharmacology* 171(2003):36–46.

75 New England Journal of Medicine: Samaha FF, et al. "A low-carbohydrate as compared with a low-fat diet in severe obesity." *New England Journal of Medicine* 348(2003):2074–81.

75 *heralded the findings*: Craig O and R Matthews. "Praise the lard." *Sunday Telegraph* (London) 25 May 2003; Atkins Nutritionals, Inc. "Let's set the record straight." <http://atkins.com/Archive/2003/5/29-77313.html>.

75 *started out eating*: "Trends in intake of energy and macronutrients—United States, 1971–2000." *Morbidity and Mortality Weekly Report* 53(2004):80–2.

75 *at the end*: Samaha FF, et al. "A low-carbohydrate as compared with a low-fat diet in severe obesity." *New England Journal of Medicine* 348(2003):2074–81.

75 *34% calories from fat*: Stern L, et al. "The effects of low-carbohydrate versus

conventional weight loss diets in severely obese adults: One-year follow-up of a randomized trial." *Annals of Internal Medicine* 140(2004):778–85.

75   *"Atkins professionals"*: Atkins Nutritionals, Inc. Commentary. "The following information was written by Atkins professionals." <http://atkins.com/Archive/2004/5/19-393409.html>.

76   *provided no weight loss advantage*: Stern L, et al. "The effects of low-carbohydrate versus conventional weight loss diets in severely obese adults: One-year follow-up of a randomized trial." *Annals of Internal Medicine* 140(2004):778–85.

76   *low-fat diets seemed to win*: Fleming RM. "The effect of high-, moderate-, and low-fat diets on weight loss and cardiovascular disease risk factors." *Preventive Cardiology* 5(2002):110–8; Dansinger ML, et al. "One year effectiveness of the Atkins, Ornish, Weight Watchers, and Zone diets in decreasing body weight and heart disease risk." Presented at the American Heart Association Scientific Sessions November 12, 2003 in Orlando, Florida.

76   *lasted at most a few months*: Bailes JR, et al. "Effect of low-carbohydrate, unlimited calorie diet on the treatment of childhood obesity: A prospective controlled study." *Metabolic Syndrome and Related Disorders* 1(2003):221–5; Boden G, et al. "Effects of the Atkins Diet in type 2 diabetes: Metabolic balance studies." 64th session of the American Diabetes Association, #321-OR, 8 June 2004; Goldstein T, et al. "Influence of a modified Atkins Diet on weight loss and glucose metabolism in obese type 2 diabetic patients." *Israel Medical Association Journal* 6(2004):314; Greene, et al. "Pilot 12-week feeding weight-loss comparison: Low-fat vs. low-carbohydrate (ketogenic) diets." Abstract presented at the North American Association for the Study of Obesity Annual Meeting 2003, *Obesity Research* 11S(2003):95OR; Greene PJ, Devecis J, and WC Willett. "Effects of low-fat vs. ultra-low-carbohydrate weight-loss diets: A 12-week pilot feeding study." Abstract presented at Nutrition Week 2004, 9–12 February 2004, in Las Vegas, Nevada; Gutierrez M, et al. "Utility of a short-term 25% carbohydrate diet on improving glycemic control in type 2 diabetes mellitus." *Journal of the American College of Nutrition* 17(1998):595–600; Meckling KA, O'Sullivan C, and D Saan. "Compoarison of a low-fat diet to a low-carbohydrate diet on weight loss, body composition, and risk factors for diabetes and cardiovascular disease in free-living, overweight men and women." *Journal of Clinical Endocrinology and Metabolism* 89(2004):2717; Nickols-Richardson, SM, Volpe JJ, and MD Coleman. "Premenopausal women following a low-carbohydrate/high-protein diet experience greater weight loss and less hunger compared to a high-carbohydrate/low-fat diet." Abstract presented at FASEB Meeting on Experimental Biology: Translating the Genome, Washington, D.C., 17–21 April 2004; Sharman MJ, et al. "Very low-carbohydrate and low-fat diets affect fasting lipids and postprandial lipemia differently in overweight men." *Journal of Nutrition* 134(2004):880–5; Sharman MJ, et al. "A ketogenic diet favorably affects serum biomarkers for cardiovascular disease in normal-weight men." *Journal of Nutrition.* 132(2002):1879–85; Sondike SB, Copperman N, and MS Jacobson. "Effects of a low-carbohydrate diet on weight loss and cardiovascular risk factor in overweight adolescents." *Journal of Pediatrics* 142(2003):253–8; Stadler DD, et al.

"Impact of 42-Day Atkins Diet and energy-matched low-fat diet on weight and anthropometric indices," *FASEB Journal* 17(4–5): Abstract of the 12th Annual FASEB Meeting on Experimental Biology: Translating the Genome, San Diego, California, 11–15 April 2003: Abstract No 453.3; Volek JS, Gomez AL, and WJ Kraemer. "Fasting lipoprotein and postprandial triacylglycerol responses to a low-carbohydrate diet supplemented with n-3 fatty acids." *Journal of the American College of Nutrition* 19(2000):383–91; Volek JS, et al. "Comparison of a very low-carbohydrate and low-fat diet on fasting lipids, LDL subclasses, insulin resistance, and postprandial lipemic responses in overweight women." *Journal of the American College of Nutrition* 23(2004):177–84; Volek JS, et al. "Body composition and hormonal responses to a carbohydrate-restricted diet." *Metabolism* 51(2002):864–70; Volek JS, et al. "An isoenergetic very low carbohydrate diet improves serum HDL cholesterol and triacylglycerol concentrations, the total cholesterol to HDL cholesterol ratio and postprandial glycemic responses compared with a low fat diet in normal weight, normolipidemic women." *Journal of Nutrition* 133(2003):2756–61; Yancy WS, Foy ME, and EC Westman. "A low-carbohydrate, ketogenic diet for type 2 diabetes mellitus." *Journal of General Internal Medicine* 19(2004):110S; Yancy YS, et al. "A pilot trial of a low-carbohydrate, ketogenic diet in patients with type 2 diabetes." *Metabolic Syndrome and Related Disorders* 1(2003):239–43.

76 *had 15 or fewer people*: Boden, G, et al. "Effects of the Atkins Diet in type 2 diabetes: Metabolic balance studies." 64th session of the American Diabetes Association, #321-OR, 8 June 2004; Greene, P, et al. "Pilot 12-week feeding weight-loss comparison: Low-fat vs. low-carbohydrate (ketogenic) diets." Abstract presented at the North American Association for the Study of Obesity annual meeting 2003, *Obesity Research* 11S(2003):95OR; Greene, PJ, Devecis J, and WC Willett. "Effects of low-fat vs. ultra-low-carbohydrate weight-loss diets: A 12-week pilot feeding study." Abstract presented at Nutrition Week 2004, February 9–12, 2004, in Las Vegas, Nevada; Kossoff EH, et al. "Efficacy of the Catkins Diet as therapy for intractable epilepsy." *Neurology* 61(2003):1789–91; *Journal of Clinical Endocrinology and Metabolism* 89(2004):2717; Nickols-Richardson, SM, Volpe JJ, and MD Coleman. "Premenopausal women following a low-carbohydrate/high-protein diet experience greater weight loss and less hunger compared to a high-carbohydrate/low-fat diet." Abstract presented at FASEB Meeting on Experimental Biology: Translating the Genome, Washington, D.C., 17–21 April 2004; Sharman MJ, et al. "Very low-carbohydrate and low-fat diets affect fasting lipids and postprandial lipemia differently in overweight men." *Journal of Nutrition* 134(2004):880–5; Sharman MJ, et al. "A ketogenic diet favorably affects serum biomarkers for cardiovascular disease in normal-weight men." *Journal of Nutrition.* 132(2002):1879–85; Stadler DD, et al. "Impact of 42-Day Atkins Diet and energy-matched low-fat diet on weight and anthropometric indices," *FASEB Journal* 17(4–5): Abstract of the 12th Annual FASEB Meeting on Experimental Biology: Translating the Genome, San Diego, California, 11–15 April 2003: Abstract No 453.3; Vernon MC, et al. "Clinical experience of a carbohydrate-restricted diet: Effect on diabetes mellitus." *Metabolic Syndrome and Related Disorders* 1(2003):233–7; Volek JS, Gomez AL, and WJ Kraemer. "Fasting lipoprotein and postprandial triacylglycerol responses to a low-carbohydrate

diet supplemented with n-3 fatty acids." *Journal of the American College of Nutrition* 19(2000):383–91; Volek JS, et al. "Comparison of a very low-carbohydrate and low-fat diet on fasting lipids, LDL subclasses, insulin resistance, and postprandial lipemic responses in overweight women." *Journal of the American College of Nutrition* 23(2004):177–84; Volek JS, et al. "Body composition and hormonal responses to a carbohydrate-restricted diet." *Metabolism* 51(2002):864–70; Volek JS, et al. "An isoenergetic very low carbohydrate diet improves serum HDL cholesterol and triacylglycerol concentrations, the total cholesterol to HDL cholesterol ratio and postprandial glycemic responses compared with a low fat diet in normal weight, normolipidemic women." *Journal of Nutrition* 133(2003):2756–61; Westman EC, et al. "A pilot study of a low-carbohydrate, ketogenic diet for obesity-related polycystic ovary syndrome." *Journal of General Internal Medicine* 19(2004):111S; Yancy WS Jr, Provenzale D, and EC Westman. "Improvement of gastroesophageal reflux disease after initiation of a low-carbohydrate diet: Five brief case reports," *Alternative Therapies in Health and Medicine* 7(2001):116–9.; Yancy YS, et al. "A pilot trial of a low-carbohydrate, ketogenic diet in patients with type 2 diabetes." *Metabolic Syndrome and Related Disorders* 1(2003):239–43.

76   *lacked any control group*: Boden, G, et al. "Effects of the Atkins Diet in type 2 diabetes: Metabolic balance studies." 64th session of the American Diabetes Association, #321-OR, 8 June 2004; Hays JH, et al. "Effect of a high saturated fat and no-starch diet on serum lipid subfractions in patients with documented atherosclerotic cardiovascular disease." *Mayo Clinic Proceedings* 78(2003):1331–1336; Hickey JT. "Clinical use of a carbohydrate-restricted diet to treat the dyslipidemia of the metabolic syndrome." *Metabolic Syndrome and Related Disorders* 1(2003): 227–232; Kossoff EH, et al. "Efficacy of the Atkins Diet as therapy for intractable epilepsy." *Neurology* 61(2003):1789–91; Vernon MC, et al. "Clinical experience of a carbohydrate-restricted diet: Effect on diabetes mellitus." *Metabolic Syndrome and Related Disorders* 1(2003):233–7; Volek JS, Gomez AL, and WJ Kraemer. "Fasting lipoprotein and postprandial triacylglycerol responses to a low-carbohydrate diet supplemented with n-3 fatty acids." *Journal of the American College of Nutrition* 19(2000):383–91; Westman EC, et al. "Effect of 6-month adherence to a very low carbohydrate diet program." *American Journal of Medicine* 113(2002):30–6; Westman EC, et al. "A pilot study of a low-carbohydrate, ketogenic diet for obesity-related polycystic ovary syndrome." *Journal of General Internal Medicine* 19(2004):111S; Yancy WS, Foy ME, and EC Westman. "A low-carbohydrate, ketogenic diet for type 2 diabetes mellitus." *Journal of General Internal Medicine* 19(2004):110S; Yancy YS, et al. "A pilot trial of a low-carbohydrate, ketogenic diet in patients with type 2 diabetes." *Metabolic Syndrome and Related Disorders* 1(2003):239–43; Yancy WS Jr, Provenzale D, and EC Westman. "Improvement of gastroesophageal reflux disease after initiation of a low-carbohydrate diet: Five brief case reports," *Alternative Therapies in Health and Medicine* 7(2001):116–9.

76   *between 29% and 35% calories*: Brehm BJ, et al. "A randomized trial comparing a very low carbohydrate diet and a calorie-restricted low fat diet on body weight and cardiovascular risk factors in healthy women." *Journal of Clinical Endocrinology and Metabolism* 88(2003):1617–23; Goldstein T, et al. "Influ-

ence of a modified Atkins Diet on weight loss and glucose metabolism in obese type 2 diabetic patients." *Israel Medical Association Journal* 6(2004):314; Greene P, et al. "Pilot 12-week feeding weight-loss comparison: Low-fat vs. low-carbohydrate (ketogenic) diets." Abstract presented at the North American Association for the Study of Obesity Annual Meeting 2003, *Obesity Research* 11S(2003):95OR; Greene PJ, Devecis J, and WC Willett. "Effects of low-fat vs. ultra-low-carbohydrate weight-loss diets: A 12-week pilot feeding study." Abstract presented at Nutrition Week 2004, 9–12 February 2004, in Las Vegas, Nevada; O'Brien KD, Brehm BJ, Seeley RJ. "Greater reduction in inflammatory markers with a low-carbohydrate diet than with a calorically matched low-fat diet." Presented at American Heart Association's Scientific Sessions 2002 on November 19, 2002, Abstract ID: 117597; Samaha FF, et al. "A low-carbohydrate as compared with a low-fat diet in severe obesity." *New England Journal of Medicine* 348(2003):2074–81; Stern L, et al. "The effects of low-carbohydrate versus conventional weight loss diets in severely obese adults: One-year follow-up of a randomized trial." *Annals of Internal Medicine* 140(2004):778–85; Yancy WS Jr, et al. "A low-carbohydrate, ketogenic diet versus a low-fat diet to treat obesity and hyperlipidemia: A randomized, controlled trial." *Annals of Internal Medicine* 140(2004):769–77.

76   *not a low-fat diet*: Kennedy ET, et al. "Popular diets: Correlation to health, nutrition and obesity." *Journal of the American Dietetic Association* 101(2001):411–20.

76   *moderate-fat (30%)*: Ibid.

76   *consistent history of failure*: Braunwald E, ed. *Harrison's Advances in Cardiology*. McGraw Hill, 2002.

76   *failed to outperform*: Dansinger ML, et al. "One year effectiveness of the Atkins, Ornish, Weight Watchers, and Zone diets in decreasing body weight and heart disease risk." Presented at the American Heart Association Scientific Sessions November 12, 2003 in Orlando, Florida; Foster GD, et al. "A randomized trial of a low-carbohydrate diet for obesity." *New England Journal of Medicine* 348(2003):2082–90; Stern L, et al. "The effects of low-carbohydrate versus conventional weight loss diets in severely obese adults: One-year follow-up of a randomized trial." *Annals of Internal Medicine* 140(2004):778–85; Fleming RM. "The effect of high-, moderate-, and low-fat diets on weight loss and cardiovascular disease risk factors." *Preventive Cardiology* 5(2002):110–8.

76   *based on a study*: Gorman C. "The secrets of their success: Shedding pounds isn't easy. Keeping them off is harder still. What we can learn from those who did." *Time Magazine* 7 June 2004:107.

76   *kept it off*: Wing RR and JO Hill. "Successful weight loss maintenance." *Annual Review of Nutrition* 21(2001):323.

76   *Almost nobody's*: Fumento M. "Big fat fake: The Atkins Diet controversy and the sorry state of science journalism." *Reason* March 2003.

77   *2002 or later*: Atkins Nutritionals, Inc. "References 1–529" <http://www.AtkinsExposed.org/atkins/58/References_1_-_529.htm>.

77   *consistent since 1972*: Atkins Nutritionals, Inc. News release January 2004.

77   *nothing in the earlier books*: Atkins Nutritionals, Inc. "Frequently asked questions." <http://atkins.com/helpatkins/newfaq/answers/WhyDidDrAtkinsReviseHisNewDietRevolutionDoes.html>.

77   *medical authorities*: "Expert opinions on Atkins." <http://www.AtkinsExposed.org/atkins/22/Opinions.htm>.

78   *Typical Induction Menu*: Physicians Committee for Responsible Medicine. "Health advisory." <http://www.atkinsdietalert.org/advisory.html>.

78   *Tufts University*: "Is it possible to follow the Atkins Diet healthfully?" *Tufts University Health and Nutrition Letter* December 2003:4–5.

78   Journal of the American College of Nutrition: Anderson: JW, Konz EC, and DJA Jenkins. "Health advantages and disadvantages of weight-reducing diets: A computer analysis and critical review." *Journal of the American College of Nutrition* 19(2000):578–90.

78   Journal of the American College of Cardiology: Kappagoda CT, Hyson DA, and EA Amsterdam. "Low-carbohydrate-high-protein diets: Is there a place for them in clinical cardiology?" *Journal of the American College of Cardiology* 43(2004):725–30.

78   minimum *recommended*: American College of Gastroenterology. "American Gastroenterological Association medical position statement: Impact of dietary fiber on colon cancer occurrence." *Gastroenterology* 118(2000):1233–4.

78   *FDA's Daily Value*: U.S. Food and Drug Administration Center for Food Safety and Applied Nutrition Guidance. "How to understand and use the nutrition facts panel on food labels." Updated July 2003. <http://www.cfsan.fda.gov/~dms/foodlab.html>.

78   *Institute of Medicine*: Institute of Medicine. *Dietary Reference Intakes: Energy, Carbohydrate, Fiber, Fat, Fatty Acids, Cholesterol, Protein, and Amino Acids.* National Academy Press, September 2002.

79   *Don't Even Think*: Atkins RC. *Dr. Atkins' New Diet Revolution.* Perennial Currents, 2002:301.

79   *fewer than 3 servings*: Anderson JW, Konz EC, and DJA Jenkins. "Health advantages and disadvantages of weight-reducing diets: A computer analysis and critical review." *Journal of the American College of Nutrition* 19(2000):578–90.

79   *lowest in fiber*: Ibid.

79   *minimum daily recommendation*: American College of Gastroenterology. "American Gastroenterological Association medical position statement: Impact of dietary fiber on colon cancer occurrence." *Gastroenterology* 118(2000):1233–4.

79   *70% of the patients*: Yancy WS Jr, et al. "A low-carbohydrate, ketogenic diet versus a low-fat diet to treat obesity and hyperlipidemia: A randomized, controlled trial." *Annals of Internal Medicine* 140(2004):769–77.

79   *Atkins himself even admitted*: Recorded personal communication with John McDougall, MD on KRSO radio, Santa Rosa, CA.

80   *most comprehensive report*: "International panel of experts meets to produce world's most comprehensive, influential diet-cancer report." *Charity Wire* 13 May 2003.

80   *number one recommendation*: American Institute for Cancer Research/ World Cancer Research. *Fund Expert Report, Food, Nutrition, and the Prevention of Cancer: A Global Perspective*, 1997.

80   *limiting the consumption*: World Health Organization. "World health assembly

raises global public health to new level." <http://www.who.int/mediacentre/releases/2004/wha4/en/>.

80 *increasing the consumption*: World Health Organization. "Frequently asked questions about the WHO global strategy on diet, physical activity and health." <http://www.who.int/dietphysicalactivity/faq/en/>.

80 *very little evidence*: Atkins Nutritionals, Inc. "Live chat—Dr. Atkins on diet and cancer." 2 August 2001. <http://atkins.com/Archive/2001/12/27-219167.html>.

81 *On your official website*: Atkins Nutritionals, Inc. "New thinking on colorectal cancer, part 2." <http://atkins.com/Archive/2002/3/19-622090.html>.

81 *American Cancer Society*: American Cancer Society. "American Cancer Society guidelines on diet and cancer prevention." 9 October 1997.

81 *"preponderance" of evidence*: Kushi L and E Giovannucci. "Dietary fat and cancer." *American Journal of Medicine* 113(2002):63S-70S.

81 *consensus statement*: "Dietary fat consensus statements." *American Journal of Medicine* 113(2002):5S–8S.

81 *only review since*: September 19, 2004 Medline search of ((colorectal cancer.mp or Colorectal Neoplasms/) and (Meat/ or red meat.mp.)) limited to "review articles" published in 2003 or 2004.

81 *National Cancer Institute*: Key TJ, et al. "Diet, nutrition and the prevention of cancer." *Public Health Nutrition* 7(2004):187–200.

81 *Atkins is the ideal way*: Atkins Nutritionals, Inc. "Food and breast cancer: What's the connection? Part 2." <http://atkins.com/Archive/2002/2/14-761333.html>.

81 *automatically lowers your risk*: Ibid.

81 *half cup of lard's*: U.S. Department of Agriculture, Agricultural Research Service 2004. USDA National Nutrient Database for Standard Reference, Release 17, Nutrient Data Laboratory home page. <http://www.nal.usda.gov/fnic/foodcomp>; Anderson JW, Konz EC, and DJA Jenkins. "Health advantages and disadvantages of weight-reducing diets: A computer analysis and critical review." *Journal of the American College of Nutrition* 19(2000):578–90.

81 *Your website claims*: Atkins Nutritionals, Inc. "Food and breast cancer: What's the connection?" <http://atkins.com/Archive/2002/2/7-197330.html>.

82 *doesn't address the topic*: Kohlmeier L and M Mendez. "Controversies surrounding diet and breast cancer." *Proceedings of the Nutrition Society* 56(1997):369–82.

82 *most accurate*: Atkins Nutritionals, Inc. "Say *what*? Minding the media." <http://atkins.com/Archive/2003/7/22-983171.html>.

82 *thousands of studies*: "International panel of experts meets to produce world's most comprehensive, influential diet-cancer report." *Charity Wire* 13 May 2003.

82 *linked to breast cancer*: American Institute for Cancer Research/ World Cancer Research. *Fund Expert Report, Food, Nutrition, and the Prevention of Cancer: A Global Perspective*, 1997.

82 *re-review of the topic*: Richter WO. "Fatty acids and breast cancer—is there a relationship?" *European Journal of Medical Research* 8(2003):373–80.

82 *yet another*: Boyd NF, et al. "Dietary fat and breast cancer risk revisited: A meta-analysis of the published literature." *British Journal of Cancer* 89(2003):1672–85; Howe GR, et al. "Dietary factors and risk of breast cancer: Combined analysis of 12 case-control studies." *Journal of the National Cancer Institute* 82(1990):561–9.

82 *increased risk of breast cancer*: Saadatian-Elahi M. "Biomarkers of dietary fatty acid intake and the risk of breast cancer: A meta-analysis." *International Journal of Cancer* 111(2004):584–91.

82 *fat related to cancer*: Atkins Nutritionals, Inc. "Live chat—Dr. Atkins on diet and cancer." 2 August 2001 <http://atkins.com/Archive/2001/12/27-219167.html>.

82 *cancers of the breast*: Bingham SA. "Are imprecise methods obscuring a relation between fat and breast cancer?" *The Lancet* 362(2003):212.

82 *prostate*: Bairati I, et al. "Dietary fat and advanced prostate cancer." *Journal of Urology* 159(1998):1271–5.

82 *endometrium*: Potischman N, et al. "Dietary associations in a case-control study of endometrial cancer." *Cancer Causes and Control* 4(1993):239–50.

82 *lung*: Alavanja MC, et al. "Saturated fat intake and lung cancer risk among nonsmoking women in Missouri." *Journal of the National Cancer Institute* 85(1993):1906–16.

82 *pancreas*: Stolzenberg-Solomon RZ, et al. "Prospective study of diet and pancreatic cancer in male smokers." *American Journal of Epidemiology* 155(2002):783–92.

82 *comes from animal products*: "Revealing trans fats." *FDA Consumer* September–October 2003. Pub No FDA04-1329C.

82 *burger*: U.S. Department of Agriculture, Agricultural Research Service. USDA National Nutrient Database for Standard Reference. "Fat and fatty acid content of selected foods containing trans-fatty acids." 2004.

82 *cheese*: Ibid.

83 *butter*: "Trans fatty acids." General Conference Nutrition Council Position Statement Andrews University Nutrition Department 7 March 2002.

83 *Hot dog and turkey*: U.S. Department of Agriculture, Agricultural Research Service. USDA National Nutrient Database for Standard Reference. "Fat and fatty acid content of selected foods containing trans-fatty acids." 2004.

83 *most prestigious*: "A new academy member Center's Robert Eisenman joins Hartwell, Thomas in nation's most prestigious scientific organization." *Fred Hutchinson Cancer Research Center News* 4(1998).

83 *any incremental increase*: National Academy of Sciences Institute of Medicine. *Dietary Reference Intakes for Energy, Carbohydrate, Fiber, Fat, Fatty Acids, Cholesterol, Protein, and Amino Acids (Macronutrients)*. National Academy Press, 2002.

83 *only on science*: Fox M. "Report recommends limiting trans-fats in diet." Reuters 10 July 2002.

83 *as low as possible*: National Academy of Sciences Institute of Medicine. *Dietary Reference Intakes for Energy, Carbohydrate, Fiber, Fat, Fatty Acids, Cholesterol, Protein, and Amino Acids (Macronutrients)*. National Academy Press, 2002.

83   *accomplish neither*: Anderson JW, Konz EC, and DJA Jenkins. "Health advantages and disadvantages of weight-reducing diets: A computer analysis and critical review." *Journal of the American College of Nutrition* 19(2000):578–90.

83   *killer since the 1930s*: Atkins Nutritionals, Inc. "Trans fats heat up." <http://atkins.com/Archive/2003/7/31-167227.html>.

83   *unlimited*: Atkins RC. *Dr. Atkins' Diet Revolution.* David McKay Company, Inc., 1972:137.

83   *most concentrated source.* "Top 10 foods with trans fats." <http://my.webmd.com/content/article/70/81100.htm>.

83   *"pioneer" and an "innovator"*: Atkins Nutritionals, Inc. "The trailblazing work of Dr. Atkins." <http://atkins.com/Archive/2004/6/30-185426.html>.

83   *finally took a position*: Atkins Nutritionals, Inc. "The trailblazing work of Dr. Atkins (Part 2)." <http://atkins.com/Archive/2004/8/10-529410.html>.

84   *75% greater risk*: Cho E, et al. "Premenopausal fat intake and risk of breast cancer." *Journal of the National Cancer Institute* 95(2003):1079–85.

84   *"right kinds of dietary fat"*: *International Journal of Cancer* 111(2004):584.

84   *increased risk of breast cancer*: Cho E, et al. "Premenopausal fat intake and risk of breast cancer." *Journal of the National Cancer Institute* 95(2003):1079–85.

84   *double their breast cancer risk*: Bingham SA. "Are imprecise methods obscuring a relation between fat and breast cancer?" *The Lancet* 362(2003):212.

84   *67 grams of saturated fat*: *FASEB Journal* 17(4–5): Abstract of the 12th Annual FASEB Meeting on Experimental Biology: Translating the Genome, San Diego, California, 11–15 April 2003: Abstract No 3321.

85   *What is the relationship*: Atkins Nutritionals, Inc. "Live chat—Dr. Atkins on diet and cancer." 2 August 2001 <http://atkins.com/Archive/2001/12/27-219167.html>.

85   *brain tumors*: Kaplan S, Novikov I, and B Modan. "Nutritional factors in the etiology of brain tumors: Potential role of nitrosamines, fat, and cholesterol." *American Journal of Epidemiology* 146(1997):832–41.

85   *breast cancer*: Sieri S, et al. "Fat and protein intake and subsequent breast cancer risk in postmenopausal women." *Nutrition and Cancer* 42(2002):10–7.

85   *pancreatic cancer*: Nishi M. "Pancreas cancer." *Japanese Journal of Cancer and Chemotherapy* 28(2001):159–62.

85   *stomach cancer*: Palli D, et al. "Red meat, family history, and increased risk of gastric cancer with microsatellite instability." *Cancer Research* 61(2001):5415–9.

85   *endometrial cancer*: Shu XO, et al. "A population-based case-control study of dietary factors and endometrial cancer in Shanghai, People's Republic of China." *American Journal of Epidemiology* 137(1993):155–65.

85   *kidney cancer*: Chow WH, et al. "Protein intake and risk of renal cell cancer." *Journal of the National Cancer Institute* 86(1994):1131–9.

85   *laryngeal cancer*: Bosetti C, et al. "Energy, macronutrients and laryngeal cancer risk." *Annals of Oncology* 14(2003):907–12.

85   *esophageal cancer*: Wolfgarten E, et al. "Coincidence of nutritional habits and esophageal cancer in Germany." *Onkologie* 24(2001):546–51.

85   *lung cancer*: Sankaranarayanan R, et al. "A case-control study of diet and lung cancer in Kerala, south India." *International Journal of Cancer* 58(1994):644–9.

85   *"aggressive"*: O'Keefe SJ, et al. "Rarity of colon cancer in Africans is associated with low animal product consumption, not fiber." *American Journal of Gastroenterology* 94(1999):1373–80.

85   *single investigation described*: Atkins Nutritionals, Inc. "Doesn't a high-fat diet increase cancer risk?" <http://atkins.com/helpatkins/newfaq/answers/DoesnTAHighFatDietIncreaseCancerRisk.html>.

85   *You claim that the findings*: Ibid.

85   *official account*: "This is the outcome of the European Conference on Nutrition and Cancer held in Lyon, France on 21–24 June.…" *World Health Organization International Agency for Research on Cancer Nutrition and Lifestyle: Opportunities for Cancer Prevention.* IARC Scientific Publications No 156, 2002.

85   *500,000 individuals*: Atkins Nutritionals, Inc. "Live chat—Dr. Atkins on diet and cancer." <http://atkins.com/Archive/2001/12/27-219167.html>.

86   *at least 34 case-control*: Riboli, E. "Meat, processed meat, and colorectal cancer." Abstract of the European Conference on Nutrition and Cancer, International Agency for Research on Cancer and Europe Against Cancer, Programme of the European Commission, Abstract No 0.08, Lyon, France 21–24 June 2001.

86   *"very preliminary"*: "Colorectal cancer: Consumption of processed meat increases cancer risk." *Health and Medicine Week* 23 July 2001:12–3.

86   *interpreted with caution*: Riboli E. "Meat, processed meat, and colorectal cancer." Abstract of the European Conference on Nutrition and Cancer, International Agency for Research on Cancer and Europe Against Cancer, Programme of the European Commission, Abstract No 0.08, Lyon, France 21–24 June 2001.

86   *50% greater risk*: "Colorectal cancer: Consumption of processed meat increases cancer risk." *Health and Medicine Week* 23 July 2001:12–3.

86   *one jumbo hot dog*: U.S. Department of Agriculture, Agricultural Research Service 2004. USDA National Nutrient Database for Standard Reference, Release 17, Nutrient Data Laboratory home page. <http://www.nal.usda.gov/fnic/foodcomp>.

86   *independent review*: Norat T, et al. "Meat consumption and colorectal cancer risk." Abstract for the European Conference on Nutrition and Cancer, International Agency for Research on Cancer and Europe Against Cancer Programme of the European Commission, Abstract No 8.14, Lyon, France 21–24 June 2001.

86   *2004 review*: Key TJ, et al. "Diet, nutrition and the prevention of cancer." *Public Health Nutrition* 7(2004):187–200.

87   *single teaspoon*: U.S. Department of Agriculture, Agricultural Research Service 2004. USDA National Nutrient Database for Standard Reference, Release 17, Nutrient Data Laboratory home page. <http://www.nal.usda.gov/fnic/foodcomp>.

87   *over twice the risk*: World Health Organization. *International Agency for Research on Cancer Nutrition and Lifestyle: Opportunities for Cancer Prevention.* IARC Scientific Publications No 156, 2002:552.

87   *as much as smoking*: Ross E. "Red meat could be as carcinogenic as tobacco." *South Coast Today* 24 June 2001.

87   *official account*: World Health Organization. *International Agency for Research*

on Cancer Nutrition and Lifestyle: Opportunities for Cancer Prevention. IARC
Scientific Publications No 156, 2002:93.

87 *cut their risk*: Ibid:351.

87 *numerous cancers*: Willett WC and D Trichopoulos. "Nutrition and cancer: A
summary of the evidence." *Cancer Causes and Control* 7(1996):178.

87 *reduce heart disease mortality*: Key TJ, et al. "Dietary habits and mortality in
11,000 vegetarians and health conscious people: Results of a 17 year follow
up." *British Medical Journal* 313(1996):775–9.

87 *"somewhat risky"*: "Is it possible to follow the Atkins Diet healthfully?" *Tufts
University Health and Nutrition Letter* December 2003:4–5.

87 *another myth*: Atkins Nutritionals, Inc. "Talking about Atkins to your doctor."
<http://atkins.com/Archive/2002/6/17-1515.html>. Accessed 1 October 2004.

88 *increases calcium loss*: Ginty F. "Dietary protein and bone health." *Proceedings
of the Nutrition Society* 62(2003):867–76.

88 *Human Vitamin and Mineral Requirements*: World Health Organization and
the Food and Agriculture Organization of the United Nations. *Human Vitamin and Mineral Requirements*. Report of a joint FAO/WHO expert consultation Rome, 2002.

88 *140 grams*: 145.6 grams of protein (*Journal of the American College of Nutrition* 19(2000):578) minus 5 grams of plant protein contained in 3 cups of
salad (U.S. Department of Agriculture, Agricultural Research Service 2004.
USDA National Nutrient Database for Standard Reference, Release 17, Nutrient Data Laboratory home page. <http://www.nal.usda.gov/fnic/foodcomp>).

89 *significantly increased fracture risk*: Feskanich D, et al. "Protein consumption
and bone fractures in women." *American Journal of Epidemiology*
143(1996):472–9.

89 *Nurses' Study*: Ibid.

89 *investigators concluded*: Sellmeyer DE, et al. "A high ratio of dietary animal to
vegetable protein increases the rate of bone loss and the risk of fracture in
postmenopausal women." *American Journal of Clinical Nutrition*
73(2001):118–22.

89 *dieters doubled their risk*: Meyer HE, et al. "Dietary factors and the incidence
of hip fracture in middle-aged Norwegians. A prospective study." *American
Journal of Epidemiology* 145(1997):117–23.

89 *15 "selected" studies*: Atkins Nutritionals, Inc. "A controlled carbohydrate diet
does not negatively affect normal calcium and bone metabolism."
<http://atkins.com/science/principles/goodhealth/principleAcontrolledcarbo-
hydratedietcalciumandbone.html>.

89 *50% of bone tissue*: Ginty F. "Dietary protein and bone health." *Proceedings of
the Nutrition Society* 62(2003):867–76.

89 *less bone loss*: Hannan MT, et al. "Effect of dietary protein on bone loss in elderly men and women: The Framingham Osteoporosis Study." *Journal of Bone
and Mineral Research* 15(2000):2504–12.

89 *or fracture risk*: Munger RG, Cerhan JR, and BC Chiu. "Prospective study of
dietary protein intake and risk of hip fracture in postmenopausal women."
American Journal of Clinical Nutrition 69(1999):147–52.

89 *propensity to fall*: Nieves JW. "Calcium, vitamin D, and nutrition in elderly
adults." *Clinics in Geriatric Medicine* 19(2003):321–35.

89 *bones at risk*: Feskanich D, et al. "Protein consumption and bone fractures in women." *American Journal of Epidemiology* 143(1996):472–9; Sellmeyer DE, et al. " A high ratio of dietary animal to vegetable protein increases the rate of bone loss and the risk of fracture in postmenopausal women." *American Journal of Clinical Nutrition* 73(2001):118–22; Meyer HE, et al. "Dietary factors and the incidence of hip fracture in middle-aged Norwegians. A prospective study." *American Journal of Epidemiology* 145(1997):117–23.

90 *mediate the effects*: Meyer HE, et al. "Dietary factors and the incidence of hip fracture in middle-aged Norwegians. A prospective study." *American Journal of Epidemiology* 145(1997):117–23.

90 *seriously deficient in calcium*: Physicians Committee for Responsible Medicine. "Health advisory." <http://www.atkinsdietalert.org/advisory.html>.

90 *fallacy*: Atkins Nutritionals, Inc. "Debunking the myths: Fact vs. fallacy, part 4." <http://atkins.com/Archive/2001/12/18-578467.html>.

90 *you will get 100%*: Ibid.

90 *estimated calcium content*: Physicians Committee for Responsible Medicine. "Health advisory." <http://www.atkinsdietalert.org/advisory.html>.

90 *less than 40%*: U.S. Food and Drug Administration Center for Food Safety and Applied Nutrition Guidance. "How to understand and use the nutrition facts panel on food labels." Updated July 2003. <http://www.cfsan.fda.gov/~dms/foodlab.html>.

90 *serious dietary shortfalls*: "Is it possible to follow the Atkins Diet healthfully?" *Tufts University Health and Nutrition Letter* December 2003:4–5.

90 *risk kidney damage*: Brenner BM, Meyer TW, and TH Hostetter. "Dietary protein intake and the progressive nature of kidney disease: The role of hemodynamically mediated glomerular injury in the pathogenesis of progressive glomerularsclerosis in aging, renal ablation, and intrinsic renal disease." *New England Journal of Medicine* 307(1982):652–9.

90 *biggest myth of all*: Atkins Nutritionals, Inc. "Debunking the myths: Fact vs. fallacy, part 4." <http://atkins.com/Archive/2001/12/18-578467.html>.

91 *only about half*: Kappagoda CT, Hyson DA, and EA Amsterdam. "Low-carbohydrate-high-protein diets: Is there a place for them in clinical cardiology?" *Journal of the American College of Cardiology* 43(2004):725–30.

91 *should more appropriately*: Atkins RC. *Dr. Atkins' New Diet Revolution*. Perennial Currents, 2002:65.

91 *156 grams of protein*: *FASEB Journal* 17(4–5): Abstract of the 12th Annual FASEB Meeting on Experimental Biology: Translating the Genome, San Diego, California, 11–15 April 2003: Abstract No 3321.

91 *over 250%*: Institute of Medicine. *Dietary Reference Intakes: Energy, Carbohydrate, Fiber, Fat, Fatty Acids, Cholesterol, Protein, and Amino Acids*. National Academy Press, September 2002.

92 *over 50%*: Anderson JW, Konz EC, and DJA Jenkins. "Health advantages and disadvantages of weight-reducing diets: A computer analysis and critical review." *Journal of the American College of Nutrition* 19(2000):578–90.

92 *happening to people's arteries*: Fleming RM. "The effect of high-protein diets on coronary blood flow." *Angiology* 51(2000):817–26.

92 *heart attack waiting to happen*: Falcone LB. "Carbs are out, protein's in as the diet pendulum swings … against the grain." *Boston Herald* 12 October 1999:37.

92 *most important risk factor*: Volek JS, and EC Westman. "Very-low-carbohy-drate weight-loss diets revisited." *Cleveland Clinic Journal of Medicine* 69(2002):849, 853, 856–8.

92 *clog so rapidly*: Fleming RM. "The effect of high-protein diets on coronary blood flow." *Angiology* 51(2000):817–26.

92 *Your claim that triglycerides*: Atkins Nutritionals, Inc. "Are triglycerides as great a heart risk as high cholesterol?" <http://atkins.com/Archive/2002/6/19-692311.html>.

92 *demonstrably false*: Grundy SM, et al. "Implications of recent clinical trials for the National Cholesterol Education Program Adult Treatment Panel III Guidelines." Endorsed by the National Heart, Lung, and Blood Institute, American College of Cardiology Foundation, and American Heart Associa-tion. *Circulation* 110(2004):227–239.

92 *single most important target*: National Institutes of Health publication 01-3305, May 2001.

92 *coordinates a coalition*: "National Heart, Lung, and Blood Institute. National Cholesterol Education Program." <http://www.nhlbi.nih.gov/about/ncep/index.htm>.

93 *primary aim of therapy*: Expert Panel on Detection, Evaluation, and Treat-ment of High Blood Cholesterol in Adults. "Executive Summary of the Third Report of the National Cholesterol Education Program (NCEP) Expert Panel on Detection, Evaluation, and Treatment of High Blood Cholesterol in Adults (Adult Treatment Panel III)." *Journal of the American Medical Association* 285(2001):2486–97.

93 *may not even be*: Gotto AM Jr. "High-density lipoprotein cholesterol and triglycerides as therapeutic targets for preventing and treating coronary artery disease." *American Heart Journal* 144(2002):S33–42.

93 *concludes one review*: Miller M. "Current perspectives on the management of hypertriglyceridemia." *American Heart Journal* 140(2000):232–40.

93 *Your website, however, claims*: "Talking about Atkins to your doctor." http://atkins.com/Archive/2002/6/17-1515.html>. Accessed 1 October 2004.

93 *Atkins-funded researchers concede*: Volek JS and SC Westman. "Very-low-car-bohydrate weight-loss diets revisited." *Cleveland Clinic Journal of Medicine* 69(2002):855–62.

94 *infiltrate rabbit arteries*: Nordestgaard BG and DB Zilversmit. "Comparison of arterial intimal clearances of LDL from diabetic and nondiabetic cholesterol-fed rabbits. Differences in intimal clearance explained by size differences." *Arteriosclerosis* 9(1989):176–83.

94 *size doesn't matter*: Kornerup K, et al. "Transvascular low-density lipoprotein transport in patients with diabetes mellitus (type 2): A noninvasive in vivo isotope technique." *Arteriosclerosis, Thrombosis and Vascular Biology* 22(2002):1168–74.

94 *over a hundred publications*: Harvard School of Public Health: Frank Sacks. <http://www.hsph.harvard.edu/faculty/FrankSacks.html>.

94 *reviewed all of the evidence*: Expert Panel on Detection, Evaluation, and Treat-ment of High Blood Cholesterol in Adults. "Executive Summary of the Third Report of the National Cholesterol Education Program (NCEP) Expert Panel on Detection, Evaluation, and Treatment of High Blood Cholesterol in Adults

(Adult Treatment Panel III)." *Journal of the American Medical Association* 285(2001):2486–97.

94 *which if any is more harmful*: Sacks FM and H Campos. "Low-density lipoprotein size and cardiovascular disease: A reappraisal." *Journal of Endocrinology and Metabolism* 10(2003):4525–32.

94 *simply isn't clinically useful*: Nissen SE. "Steven Evan Nissen, MD: A conversation with the editor. Interview by William Clifford Roberts." *American Journal of Cardiology* 94(2004):320–33.

94 *all LDL types*: Sacks FM and H Campos. "Low-density lipoprotein size and cardiovascular disease: A reappraisal." *Journal of Endocrinology and Metabolism* 10(2003):4525–32.

94 *suffer a relative increase.* Dreon DM, et al. "A very-low-fat diet is not associated with improved lipoprotein profiles in men with a predominance of large, low-density lipoproteins." *American Journal of Clinical Nutrition* 69(1999):411–8.

95 *can not only reduce*: Barnard RJ. "Effects of life-style modification on serum lipids." *Archives of Internal Medicine* 151(1991):1389–94

95 *routinely drastically improve*: Beard CM, et al. "Effects of diet and exercise on qualitative and quantitative measures of LDL and its susceptibility to oxidation." *Arteriosclerosis, Thrombosis and Vascular Biology* 16(1996):201–7.

95 *does not allow*: Volek JS and EC Westman. "Very-low-carbohydrate weight-loss diets revisited." *Cleveland Clinic Journal of Medicine* 69(2002):849, 853, 856–8.

95 *worsen so dramatically*: Fleming RM. "The effect of high-protein diets on coronary blood flow." *Angiology* 51(2000):817–26.

95 *Dr. Atkins warned*: Atkins RC. "The cholesterol drug bonanza." <http://atkins.com/Archive/2002/9/23-518825.html>.

95 *won't lower one's cholesterol enough*: Westman EC, et al. "Effect of 6-month adherence to a very low carbohydrate diet program." *American Journal of Medicine* 113(2002):30–6.

95 *seriously worsen heart disease*: Fleming RM. "The effect of high-protein diets on coronary blood flow." *Angiology* 51(2000):817–26.

95 *first line of defense*: Atkins RC. "The cholesterol drug bonanza." <http://atkins.com/Archive/2002/9/23-518825.html>.

95 *the foundation*: Expert Panel on Detection, Evaluation, and Treatment of High Blood Cholesterol in Adults. "Executive Summary of the Third Report of the National Cholesterol Education Program (NCEP) Expert Panel on Detection, Evaluation, and Treatment of High Blood Cholesterol in Adults (Adult Treatment Panel III)." *Journal of the American Medical Association* 285(2001):2486–97.

95 *reduced intakes of saturated fat*: National Institutes of Health publication 01-3305, May 2001.

95 *exactly the opposite*: Kappagoda CT, Hyson DA, and EA Amsterdam. "Low-carbohydrate-high-protein diets: Is there a place for them in clinical cardiology?" *Journal of the American College of Cardiology* 43(2004):725–30.

95 *single most important risk factor*: Expert Panel on Detection, Evaluation, and Treatment of High Blood Cholesterol in Adults. "Executive Summary of the Third Report of the National Cholesterol Education Program (NCEP) Expert

Panel on Detection, Evaluation, and Treatment of High Blood Cholesterol in Adults (Adult Treatment Panel III)." *Journal of the American Medical Association* 285(2001):2486–97.

95 *number one killer*: "National Cholesterol Education Program. Second Report of the Expert Panel on Detection, Evaluation, and Treatment of High Blood Cholesterol in Adults (Adult Treatment Panel II)." *Circulation* 89(1994):1333–445.

95 *down to double digits*: Ibid.

95 *fraction of those*: Janus ED, et al. "The modernization of Asia: Implications for coronary heart disease." *Circulation* 94(1996):2671–3.

95 *lower than 95*. Ornish D. "Statins and the soul of medicine." *American Journal of Cardiology* 89(2002):1286.

95 *may be ideal*: O'Keefe JH, et al. "Optimal low-density lipoprotein is 50 to 70 mg/dl: lower is better and physiologically normal." *Journal of the American College of Cardiology* 43(2004):2142–6.

95 *considered optimal for all individuals*: McKenney JM. "Update on the National Cholesterol Education Program Adult Treatment Panel III Guidelines: Getting to goal." *Pharmacotherapy* 23(2003):26S-33S.

95 *editor-in-chief*: Baylor University Institute for Biomedical Studies. "William C Roberts, M.D."
<http://www.baylor.edu/biomedical_studies/index.php?id=19528>.

96 *pure vegetarian*: Roberts WC. "Shifting from decreasing risk to actually preventing and arresting atherosclerosis." *American Journal of Cardiology* 83(1999):816–7.

96 *The only diet*: Lock DR, et al. "Apolipoprotein E levels in vegetarians." *Metabolism* 31(1982):917–21; Roshanai F and TA Sanders. "Assessment of fatty acid intakes in vegans and omnivores." *Human Nutrition. Applied Nutrition.* 38(1984):345–54; Fisher M, et al. "The effect of vegetarian diets on plasma lipid and platelet levels." *Archives of Internal Medicine.* 146(1986):1193–7; Thorogood M, et al. "Plasma lipids and lipoprotein cholesterol concentrations in people with different diets in Britain *British Medical Journal* (Clin Res Ed). 295(1987):351–3; Sanders TA and F Roshanai. "Platelet phospholipid fatty acid composition and function in vegans compared with age- and sex-matched omnivore controls." *European Journal of Clinical Nutrition.* 46(1992):823–31; Thomas EL, et al. "An in vivo 13C magnetic resonance spectroscopic study of the relationship between diet and adipose tissue composition. *Lipids.* 31(1996):145–51; Toohey ML, et al. "Cardiovascular disease risk factors are lower in African-American vegans compared to lacto-ovo-vegetarians." *Journal of the American College of Nutrition* 17(1998):425–34; Li D, et al. "The association of diet and thrombotic risk factors in healthy male vegetarians and meat-eaters." *European Journal of Clinical Nutrition* 53(1999):612–9; Krajcovicova-Kudlackova M, et al. "Traditional and alternative nutrition—levels of homocysteine and lipid parameters in adults." *Scandanavian Journal of Clinical Investigation* 60(2000):657–64; Fokkema MR, et al. "Short-term supplementation of low-dose gamma-linolenic acid (GLA), alpha-linolenic acid (ALA), or GLA plus ALA does not augment LCP omega 3 status of Dutch vegans to an appreciable extent." *Prostaglandins, Leukotrienes, and Essential Fatty Acids* 63(2000):287–92.

96   *best current published data*: Greenlund KJ, et al. "Trends in self-reported mul-
      tiple cardiovascular disease risk factors among adults in the United States,
      1991–1999." *Archives of Internal Medicine* 164(2004):181–8.
96   *almost every single study*: Larosa JC, et al. "Effects of high-protein, low-car-
      bohydrate dieting on plasma lipoproteins and body weight." *Journal of the
      American Dietetic Association* 77(1980):264–70; SB Lewis, et al. "Effect of
      diet composition on metabolic adaptations to hypocaloric nutrition: Com-
      parison of high carbohydrate and high fat isocaloric diets." *American Jour-
      nal of Clinical Nutrition* 30(1977):160–70; Evans E, Stock AL, and J Yudkin.
      "The absence of undesirable changes during consumption of the low carbo-
      hydrate diet." *Nutrition and Metabolism* 17(1974):360–7; Sondike SB, Cop-
      perman N, and MS Jacobson. "Effects of a low-carbohydrate diet on weight
      loss and cardiovascular risk factor in overweight adolescents." *Journal of
      Pediatrics* 142(2003):253–8; Foster GD, et al. "A randomized trial of a low-
      carbohydrate diet for obesity." *New England Journal of Medicine*
      348(2003):2082–90; Samaha FF, et al. "A low-carbohydrate as compared
      with a low-fat diet in severe obesity." *New England Journal of Medicine*
      348(2003):2074–81; Stern L, et al. "The effects of low-carbohydrate versus
      conventional weight loss diets in severely obese adults: One-year follow-up
      of a randomized trial." *Annals of Internal Medicine* 140(2004):778–85;
      Freedman MR, King J, and E Kennedy. "Popular diets: A scientific review."
      Obesity Research 9(2001):1S-40S; Sharman MJ, et al. "A ketogenic diet favor-
      ably affects serum biomarkers for cardiovascular disease in normal-weight
      men." *Journal of Nutrition* 132(2002):1879–85; Brehm BJ, et al. "A random-
      ized trial comparing a very low carbohydrate diet and a calorie-restricted
      low fat diet on body weight and cardiovascular risk factors in healthy
      women." *Journal of Clinical Endocrinology and Metabolism*
      88(2003):1617–23; Yancy WS Jr, et al. "A low-carbohydrate, ketogenic diet
      versus a low-fat diet to treat obesity and hyperlipidemia: A randomized,
      controlled trial." *Annals of Internal Medicine* 140(2004):769–77; Sharman
      MJ, et al. "Very low-carbohydrate and low-fat diets affect fasting lipids and
      postprandial lipemia differently in overweight men." *Journal of Nutrition*
      134(2004):880–5; Volek JS, et al. "An isoenergetic very low carbohydrate diet
      improves serum HDL cholesterol and triacylglycerol concentrations, the
      total cholesterol to HDL cholesterol ratio and postprandial glycemic
      responses compared with a low fat diet in normal weight, normolipidemic
      women." *Journal of Nutrition* 133(2003):2756–61.
96   *one single uncontrolled Atkins-funded study*: Westman EC, et al. "Effect of 6-
      month adherence to a very low carbohydrate diet program." *American Journal
      of Medicine* 113(2002):30–6.
96   *study of 4,587 adults*: Barnard RJ. "Effects of life-style modification on serum
      lipids." *Archives of Internal Medicine* 151(1991):1389–94.
96   *30% in 2 weeks*: Jenkins DJ, et al. "Effects of a dietary portfolio of cholesterol-
      lowering foods vs. lovastatin on serum lipids and C-reactive protein." *Journal
      of the American Medical Association* 290(2003):502–10.
96   *decreasing blood flow 40%*. Fleming RM. "The effect of high-protein diets on
      coronary blood flow." *Angiology* 51(2000):817–26.
97   *This claim is similar*: Atkins Nutritionals, Inc. "Yahoo chat—Dr. Atkins on

lowering cardiac risk factors." 16 August 2001
<http://atkins.com/Archive/2001/12/27-836486.html>.

97 *demonstrably false*: Grundy SM, et al. "Implications of recent clinical trials for
the National Cholesterol Education Program Adult Treatment Panel III
Guidelines." Endorsed by the National Heart, Lung, and Blood Institute,
American College of Cardiology Foundation, and American Heart Association. *Circulation* 110(2004):227–239.

97 *coalition of over 30 major medical*: National Heart, Lung, and Blood Institute.
National Cholesterol Education Program. Coordinating Committee Member-
ship Roster <http://www.nhlbi.nih.gov/about/ncep/ncep_ros.htm>.

97 *sufficient evidence*: McKenney JM. "Update on the National Cholesterol Education Program Adult Treatment Panel III Guidelines: Getting to goal." *Pharmacotherapy* 23(2003):26S-33S.

97 *lower the LDL level to goal*: Ibid.

97 *Atkins Diet can't do*: Westman EC, et al. "Effect of 6-month adherence to a very
low carbohydrate diet program." *American Journal of Medicine* 113(2002):30–6.

97 *has not been resolved*: National Institutes of Health publication 01-3305 May
2001.

97 *In all persons*: Expert Panel on Detection, Evaluation, and Treatment of High
Blood Cholesterol in Adults. "Executive Summary of the Third Report of the
National Cholesterol Education Program (NCEP) Expert Panel on Detection,
Evaluation, and Treatment of High Blood Cholesterol in Adults (Adult Treat-
ment Panel III)." *Journal of the American Medical Association*
285(2001):2486–97.

97 *secondary target of risk-reduction*: Ibid.

97 *more important than significantly*: McKenney JM. "Update on the National
Cholesterol Education Program Adult Treatment Panel III Guidelines: Getting to goal." *Pharmacotherapy* 23(2003):26S-33S.

98 *seriously weaken coronary artery blood flow*: Fleming RM. "The effect of high-
protein diets on coronary blood flow." *Angiology* 51(2000):817–26.

98 *Atkins does not believe*: Atkins Nutritionals, Inc. "I am just starting Atkins but
my physician says I should be on cholesterol-lowering medication. What
should I do?" <http://atkins.com/helpatkins/newfaq/answers/IAmJustStartin-
gAtkinsButMyPhysicianSaysIShould.html>.

98 *byproduct of defective protein*: Atkins Nutritionals, Inc. "Meaningful tests:
Blood lipids." <http://atkins.com/Archive/2002/5/14-516408.html>.

98 *birth defects*: McLean RR, et al."Homocysteine as a predictive factor for hip
fracture in older persons." *New England Journal of Medicine*
350(2004):2042–9.

98 *fatal blood clots*: Wald DS, Law M, and JK Morris. "Homocysteine and cardiovascular disease: Evidence on causality from a meta-analysis." *British Medical
Journal* 325(2002):1202.

98 *depression*: Tiemeier H, et al. "Vitamin B12, folate, and homocysteine in
depression: The Rotterdam Study." *American Journal of Psychiatry*
159(2002):2099–101.

98 *osteoporosis*: McLean RR, et al. "Homocysteine as a predictive factor for hip
fracture in older persons." *New England Journal of Medicine*
350(2004):2042–9.

98   *Alzheimer's Disease*: Diaz-Arrastia R. "Homocysteine and neurologic disease."
     Archives of Neurology 57(2000):1422–7.

98   *Atkins Nutritional Approach*: Atkins Nutritionals, Inc. "Homocysteine: An idea
     whose time has come." <http://atkins.com/Archive/2002/9/25-87674.html>.

98   *highly significant worsening*: Hays JH, et al. "Effect of a high saturated fat and
     no-starch diet on serum lipid subfractions in patients with documented ath-
     erosclerotic cardiovascular disease." *Mayo Clinic Proceedings* 78(2003):1331–6.

98   *homocysteine level* under *10*: Malinow MR, et al. "Homocyst(e)ine, diet, and
     cardiovascular diseases: A statement for healthcare professionals from the
     nutrition committee, American Heart Association." *Circulation*
     99(1999):178–82.

98   *Above 10 mcmol/L*: Atkins Nutritionals, Inc. "Meaningful tests: Blood lipids."
     <http://atkins.com/Archive/2002/5/14-516408.html>.

98   *related to cancer*: "Elevated homocysteine levels and increased risk of cervical
     cancer." <http://atkins.com/Archive/2002/8/23-936833.html>.

98   *concerning*: Hays JH, et al. "Effect of a high saturated fat and no-starch diet
     on serum lipid subfractions in patients with documented atherosclerotic car-
     diovascular disease." *Mayo Clinic Proceedings* 78(2003):1331–6.

99   *rise on the Atkins Diet*: Ornish D. "Was Dr. Atkins right?" *Journal of the Ameri-
     can Dietetic Association* 104(2004):537–42.

99   *fall on the vegan diet*: Fleming RM. "The effect of high-, moderate-, and low-
     fat diets on weight loss and cardiovascular disease risk factors." *Preventive
     Cardiology* 5(2002):110–8.

99   Preventive Medicine *article*: DeRose DJ, et al. "Vegan diet-based lifestyle pro-
     gram rapidly lowers homocysteine levels." *Preventive Medicine*
     30(2000):225–33.

99   *both of the two studies*: Hays JH, et al. "Effect of a high saturated fat and no-
     starch diet on serum lipid subfractions in patients with documented athero-
     sclerotic cardiovascular disease." *Mayo Clinic Proceedings* 78(2003):1331–6;
     Ornish D. "Was Dr. Atkins right?" *Journal of the American Dietetic Association*
     104(2004):537–42.

99   *Atkins also felt*: Atkins Nutritionals, Inc. "I am just starting Atkins but my
     physician says I should be on cholesterol-lowering medication. What should I
     do?" <http://atkins.com/helpatkins/newfaq/answers/IAmJustStartingAtkins-
     ButMyPhysicianSaysIShould.html>.

99   *four and one-half times*: Atkins Nutritionals, Inc. "Meaningful tests: Blood
     lipids." <http://atkins.com/Archive/2002/5/14-516408.html>.

99   *with stroke risk as well*: Hackam DG and SS Anand. "Emerging risk factors for
     atherosclerotic vascular disease: A critical review of the evidence." *Journal of
     the American Medical Association* 290(2003):932–40.

99   *strictly related to body fatness*: Bo M, et al. "Body fat is the main predictor of
     fibrinogen levels in healthy non-obese men." *Metabolism* 53(2004):984–8.

99   *ineffective in lowering CRP*: Volek JS, et al. "An isoenergetic very low carbohy-
     drate diet improves serum HDL cholesterol and triacylglycerol concentra-
     tions, the total cholesterol to HDL cholesterol ratio and postprandial
     glycemic responses compared with a low fat diet in normal weight, nor-
     molipidemic women." *Journal of Nutrition* 133(2003):2756–61; Hays JH, et al.
     "Effect of a high saturated fat and no-starch diet on serum lipid subfractions

in patients with documented atherosclerotic cardiovascular disease." *Mayo Clinic Proceedings* 78(2003):1331–6; Volek JS, et al. "Comparison of a very low-carbohydrate and low-fat diet on fasting lipids, LDL subclasses, insulin resistance, and postprandial lipemic responses in overweight women." *Journal of the American College of Nutrition* 23(2004):177–84.

99   *despite a loss of body fat*: Hays JH, et al. "Effect of a high saturated fat and no-starch diet on serum lipid subfractions in patients with documented athero-sclerotic cardiovascular disease." *Mayo Clinic Proceedings* 78(2003):1331–6.

99   *One unpublished meeting abstract*: O'Brien, KD, et al. "Greater reduction in inflammatory markers with a low-carbohydrate diet than with a calorically matched low-fat diet." Presented at American Heart Association's Scientific Sessions 19 November 2002: Abstract No 117597.

99   *two others did not*: Scheett, TP, et al. "Comparison between ketogenic and low-fat diets on high-sensitivity C-reactive protein and inflammatory cytokines in normal-weight women," *FASEB Journal* 17 (4–5), 2003: Abstract No 698.5; Ornish D. "Most weight loss, LDL reduction on Ornish Diet." <http://aolsvc.health.webmd.aol.com/content/Article/77/90389.htm>.

100   *not by the Atkins Diet*: Ornish D. "Most weight loss, LDL reduction on Ornish Diet" <http://aolsvc.health.webmd.aol.com/content/Article/77/90389.htm>.

100   *lower CRP levels 45%*: Wegge JK, et al. "Effect of diet and exercise intervention on inflammatory and adhesion molecules in postmenopausal women on hor-mone replacement therapy and at risk for coronary artery disease." *Metabo-lism* 53(2004):377–81.

100   *an average of 30%*: Jenkins DJ, et al. "Effects of a dietary portfolio of choles-terol-lowering foods vs. lovastatin on serum lipids and C-reactive protein." *Journal of the American Medical Association* 290(2003):502–10.

100   *associated with heart attack*: Hackam DG and SS Anand. "Emerging risk fac-tors for atherosclerotic vascular disease: A critical review of the evidence." *Journal of the American Medical Association* 290(2003):932–40.

100   *tends to rise*: Ornish D. "Was Dr. Atkins right?" *Journal of the American Dietetic Association* 104(2004):537–42.

100   *drop on control low-fat*: O'Keefe JH Jr, et al. "Optimal low-density lipoprotein is 50 to 70 mg/dl: Lower is better and physiologically normal." *Journal of the American College of Cardiology* 43(2004):2142–6.

100   *really bad cholesterol*: Hackam DG and SS Anand. "Emerging risk factors for atherosclerotic vascular disease: A critical review of the evidence." *Journal of the American Medical Association* 290(2003):932–40.

100   *strong risk factor*: Atkins Nutritionals, Inc. "Meaningful tests: Blood lipids." <http://atkins.com/Archive/2002/5/14-516408.html>.

100   *also tends to rise*: Ornish D. "Was Dr Atkins right?" *Journal of the American Dietetic Association* 104(2004):537–42.

100   *fall on the control vegan*: O'Keefe JH Jr, et al. "Optimal low-density lipoprotein is 50 to 70 mg/dl: Lower is better and physiologically normal." *Journal of the American College of Cardiology* 43(2004):2142–6.

101   *ridiculous*: Burros M. "Atkins diet revises message on meat, fat." *The New York Times* 18 January 2004.

101   *cancer, diabetes, and heart disease*: American Institute for Cancer Research/World Cancer Research Fund. *Food, Nutrition, and the Prevention of*

Cancer: A Global Perspective. 1997; Cho E, et al. "Premenopausal fat intake and risk of breast cancer." *Journal of the National Cancer Institute* 95(2003):1079–85; *Report of a Joint WHO/FAO Expert Consultation. Diet, Nutrition and the Prevention of Chronic Diseases.* WHO Technical Report Series 916, 2003.

101 *Trans fats act very similarly*: Davis JL. "Atkins diet goes on a diet." *Medscape Medical News* 21 January 2004.

101 *overwhelming*: Lichenstein AH and LV Horn. "Very low fat diets." *Circulation* 98(1998):935–9.

101 *2004 review*: Srinath RK and MB Katan. "Diet, nutrition and the prevention of hypertension and cardiovascular diseases." *Public Health Nutrition* 7(2004):167–86.

101 *30% of their calories: FASEB Journal* 17(4–5): Abstract of the 12th Annual FASEB Meeting on Experimental Biology: Translating the Genome, San Diego, California, 11–15 April 2003: Abstract No 3321.

101 *Framingham Nurses' Study*: Atkins Nutritionals, Inc. "Big fat lies." <http://atkins.com/Archive/2001/12/21-587266.html>.

102 *the saturated fat found*: Connor WE. "Harbingers of coronary heart disease: Dietary saturated fatty acids and cholesterol. Is chocolate benign because of its stearic acid content?" *American Journal of Clinical Nutrition* 70(1999):951–2.

102 *greater risk of coronary heart disease*: Hu FB, et al. "Dietary saturated fats and their food sources in relation to the risk of coronary heart disease in women." *American Journal of Clinical Nutrition* 70(1999):1001–8.

102 *leads to higher blood cholesterol*: Atkins Nutritionals, Inc. "Debunking the myths: Fact vs. fallacy, part 5." <http://atkins.com/Archive/2001/12/18-292461.html>.

102 *56-year history*: "A timeline of milestones from the Framingham Heart Study." <http://www.framingham.com/heart/timeline.htm>.

102 *over 1,000 scientific papers*: "The Framingham Heart Study." <http://www.framingham.com/heart/backgrnd.htm>.

102 *Director of the Framingham Cardiovascular Center*: "Affairs of the Heart." *Scientific American Frontiers* (PBS) 23 January 2001 <http://www.pbs.org/saf/1104/index.html>.

102 *Very weak science*: Personal communication to JoAnn Farb. 24 January 2000.

102 *adopted a vegetarian diet*: "Affairs of the Heart." *Scientific American Frontiers* (PBS) 23 January 2001 <http://www.pbs.org/saf/1104/index.html>.

103 *neutral or cholesterol-lowering effect*: Atkins Nutritionals, Inc. "The truth about fat." <http://atkins.com/Archive/2004/2/3-915798.html>.

103 *candy manufacturers' websites*: National Confectioners Association. "Research shows 'chocolate does not raise cholesterol.'" <http://www.candyusa.org/Media/Nutrition/chocolate_cholesterol.asp>.

103 *Hershey's corporate website*: Hershey's. "Cholesterol." <http://www.hersheys.com/nutrition_consumer/cholesterol.shtml>. Accessed 10 October 2004.

103 *Mars candy bar corporation*: Chocolate Information Center. "Stearic acid in chocolate and its neutral effect on cholesterol." <http://www.chocolateinfo.com/sr/sr_article_11.jsp>.

103   *the beef industry*: Cattlemen's Beef Board. "Nutrition."
      <http://www.beefitswhatsfordinner.com/askexpert/nutrition.asp>.

103   *do raise one's bad cholesterol*: Katan MP, Zock PR, and RP Mensink. "Effects of
      fats and fatty acids on blood lipids in humans: An overview." *Journal of the
      American College of Nutrition* 60 (1994):1017S–1022S.

103   *strongly linked with early heart attack*: Kromhout D, et al. "Dietary saturated
      and trans fatty acids and cholesterol and 25-year mortality from coronary
      heart disease: The Seven Countries Study." *Preventive Medicine*
      24(1995):308–15.

103   *even more than other saturated fats*: Hu FB, et al. "Dietary saturated fats and
      their food sources in relation to the risk of coronary heart disease in women."
      American Journal of Clinical Nutrition 70(1999):1001–8.

103   *ability to thicken the blood*: Connor WE. "Harbingers of coronary heart dis-
      ease: Dietary saturated fatty acids and cholesterol. Is chocolate benign
      because of its stearic acid content?" *American Journal of Clinical Nutrition*
      70(1999):951–2.

104   *get ripped off*: Fox M. "Low-carb fad seen as unhealthy and a ripoff." *Reuters*
      22 June 2004.